8V

G

ple q

Multiple Choice Questions in Psy

300)

Multiple Choice Questions in Psychiatry

Second Edition

Geoffrey Glew

MB, BS, MRANZCP, MRCPsych

Clinical Director, Prince Albert Psychiatric Centre,
Saskatchewan;
Chief of Psychiatry, Holy Family Hospital, Prince Albert;
Clinical Instructor, University of Saskatchewan

BUTTERWORTHS

London - Boston - Sydney - Wellington - Durban - Toronto

First published 1978
Reprinted 1978
Second edition 1981

British Library Cataloguing in Publication Data

Glew, Geoffrey
Multiple choice questions in psychiatry.–2nd ed.
1. Psychiatry–Problems, exercises, etc.
I. Title
616.89'0076 RC457

ISBN 0–407–00225–1

Typeset by Scribe Design, Gillingham, Kent
Printed in Great Britain by Redwood Burn Ltd., Trowbridge, Wiltshire.

Contents

Preface to the Second Edition

The first edition of this book was intended for candidates preparing for the Preliminary Test of the Royal College of Psychiatrists. Five papers covered basic sciences and elementary psychopathology.

In the second edition, together with the above, three papers are provided for Membership Examination candidates. Some of the new questions require familiarity with research findings. Authors' names are quoted to a much greater extent than occurs in the actual Membership Examination Multiple Choice Questions. This is a ruse to confront the student with important studies in psychiatry that may be mentioned by the examiners in the *viva*. Or the candidate may allude to them in order to appear erudite.

The reading list has been revised and enlarged.

Introduction

This collection of eight papers consists of 480 questions covering 2400 items providing practice for Multiple Choice Question examinations in psychiatry such as those held by the Royal College of Psychiatrists. Papers 1 to 5 are based on the syllabus for the Preliminary Test of the Royal College; papers 6 to 8 on the Membership Examination.

Subjects covered in papers 1 to 5 include neuroanatomy, neurophysiology, biochemistry, neuroendocrinology, action of drugs on the central nervous system, genetics, psychology, behaviour therapy, ethology, basic clinical psychopathology, statistics and epidemiology.

Papers 6 to 8 cover the management of mental illnesses including organic conditions, psychoses and neuroses. Questions are included on alcoholism, anorexia nervosa, bereavement, child psychiatry, community psychiatry, criminology, drug abuse, history of psychiatry, legal matters, leucotomy, mental retardation, psychomatic medicine, sexual disorders and suicide.

As with all large collections of multiple choice questions, it is inevitable that the face validity of some questions will be disputed. In addition, *phi* indices have not been calculated for the majority of items and their discriminatory power between better and weaker candidates can only be conjectured. It is felt, nevertheless, that this collection meets a current need.

Wording and Explanatory Notes

A number of standard terms has evolved for use in the wording of stems These include *characteristic, recognized* and *typical*.

A *characteristic* feature is one which occurs so often as, usually, to be of some diagnostic significance and, if it were not present, might lead to doubt being cast on the diagnosis.

A *recognized* feature is one that has been reported and that is a fact a candidate would reasonably be expected to know.

The term *typical* is more or less synonymous with *characteristic.*

Pathognomic and *specific* indicate features that occur in the disease named and no other.

The *majority* means at least 50%.

Each paper consists of sixty questions (five parts to each question). The time allowed for each paper is two hours.

Each question consists of an initial statement (or 'stem') followed by five possible completions (or 'items') identified by A,B,C,D,E. Each candidate should indicate whether he thinks a particular item is True or False. T = True; F = False; D = Do not know.

If he is uncertain he must mark D (= do not know). For each item correctly completed (i.e. a true statement indicated as True, or a false statement indicated as False) one mark will be gained (i.e. +1).

For each item incorrectly completed (i.e. a false statement indicated as True, or vice versa) one mark will be lost (i.e. −1).

For each item completed labelled D, no marks will be gained or lost (i.e. 0).

There is no restriction on the number of True or False items in a question. It is possible for all the items in a question to be True, or for all to be False.

Examination Technique

1. Calculate your time allowance so that half-way through the paper you can see whether you are ahead or behind.
2. If it is your plan to answer in rough in the question book and then transfer to the answer paper, allow sufficient time for the transferring.
3. Read each question carefully.
4. Leave difficult questions, mark them distinctly in the question book and return to them later.
5. If you are unsure of the answer, then only put 'don't know' if you are completely in the dark. Questions often contain clues.
6. When transferring answers from the question book to the answer paper (if this is your plan) be sure to mark the right ones. This is not as elementary as it sounds. The M.R.C.Psych. answer sheet is set out in two columns (as are the answers in this book); the logical way is to work down the left column and then the right one. In fact, one must jump from left to right and then back again.
7. Finally: don't panic!

Acknowledgement

The author is indebted to Dr. John Anderson whose practical book on Multiple Choice Questions in Medicine provided the definitions of wording used in stems. Ten questions were purloined from Dr. Anderson's collection of 150.

Reference: John Anderson, *The Multiple Choice Question in Medicine*, Pitman Medical Publishing Co Ltd, Tunbridge Wells, 1976

Reading List

Behaviour Therapy

Meyer, V. and Chesser, E. S., *Behaviour Therapy in Clinical Psychiatry*, Penguin, London, 1970

Biochemistry

McIlwain, H. and Bachelard, H. S., *Biochemistry and the Central Nervous System*, Longman, London, 1971

Clinical Psychopathology and Therapeutics

Arieti, S., *American Handbook of Psychiatry*, Second Edition, Basic Books, New York, 1974

Forrest, A., Affleck, J. and Zealley, A., *Companion to Psychiatric Studies,* Second Edition, Churchill Livingstone, Edinburgh, London & New York, 1978

Granville-Grossman, K., *Recent Advances in Clinical Psychiatry*, Number Two: 1976; Number Three: 1979, Churchill Livingstone, Edinburgh, London & New York

Kaplan, H.I., Freedman, A.M. and Sadock, B.J., *Comprehensive Textbook of Psychiatry III*, Williams & Wilkins, Baltimore, 1980

Nicholi, A.M. Jr., *The Harvard Guide to Modern Psychiatry*, Harvard University Press, Cambridge, Massachusetts and London, England, 1978

Rutter, M. and Hersov, L., *Child Psychiatry*, Blackwell Scientific Publications, Oxford, London, Edinburgh & Melbourne, 1977

Wing, J.K., *Schizophrenia. Towards a New Synthesis*, Academic Press, London, 1978

Drugs

Meyler, L. and Herxheimer, A., *Side Effects of Drugs*, Excerpta Medica, 1972

Simpson, L. L., *Drug Treatment of Mental Disorders*, Raven Press, 1976

Ethology

Lorenz, K., *Studies in Animal and Human Behaviour*, Vols. I and II, Methuen, London, 1970

Genetics

Carter, C. O., *An ABC of Medical Genetics*, The Lancet Ltd, London, 1969

Fraser, G. and Mayo, O., *Textbook of Human Genetics*, Blackwell, Oxford, 1975

Heaton-Ward, W. A., *Mental Subnormality*, John Wright & Sons, Bristol, 1975

Kirman, B. and Bicknell, J., *Mental Handicap,* Longman, London, 1975

Slater, E. and Cowie, V., *The Genetics of Mental Disorders*, Oxford University Press, 1971

Neuroanatomy and Neurophysiology

Brodal, A., *Neurological Anatomy in Relation to Clinical Medicine*, Oxford University Press, 1969

Chusid, J. G., *Correlative Neuroanatomy and Functional Neurology*, Lange, 1973

Gatz, A. J., *Clinical Neuroanatomy and Neurophysiology*, F. A. Davis Co., Bristol, 1970

Lenman, J. A. R., *Clinical Neurophysiology*, Blackwell, Oxford, 1975

Mitchell, G. A. G., *The Essentials of Neuroanatomy*, Longman, London, 1971

Psychology

Atkinson, R. A., *Contemporary Psychology: Readings from Scientific American,* W. H. Freeman & Co., Reading, 1971

Hilgard, E. R., Atkinson, R.C. and Atkinson, R.L., *Introduction to Psychology*, Harcourt Brace, New York, 1971

Statistics

Colton, T., *Statistics in Medicine,* Little, Brown & Co., Boston, Mass., 1974

Harper, W. M., *Statistics,* Macdonald & Evans, Plymouth, 1971

Mould, R. F., *Introductory Medical Statistics*, Pitman, London, 1976

Preliminary Test Questions

Paper 1

1. **The following statements are true of the vagus nerve:**
   A Its effects are blocked by acetylcholine
   B It contains sensory fibres from the pharynx and larynx
   C It innervates abdominal viscera
   D It is both efferent and afferent
   E It innervates thoracic viscera

2. **A delusion is:**
   A Never shared by another person
   B Not amenable to reason
   C A false belief
   D Recognized as silly by the patient
   E Effectively treated by behaviour therapy

3. **Recognized functions of the limbic system include:**
   A Memory
   B Spinal reflexes
   C Emotional reactions
   D Motivation
   E Conditioned reflexes

4. **Pseudo-hallucinations are recognized symptoms of:**
   A Malingering
   B Hysteria
   C Pseudo-neurotic schizophrenia
   D Bereavement
   E Schizophrenia

5. The following statements concerning schizophrenia in the general population of the United Kingdom are correct:
   A Point prevalence is greater than 0·5%
   B Prevalence is highest in Social Class V
   C The peak incidence for males occurs at over age 35 years
   D Expectancy by age 65 is greater than 0·5%
   E Incidence is less than 0·5% per year

6. Hallucinations are recognized symptoms of:
   A Obsessional neurosis
   B Depressive psychosis
   C Temporal lobe epilepsy
   D Schizophrenia
   E Atropine poisoning

7. Recognized functions of the hypothalamus include control of:
   A Balance
   B Hunger
   C Proprioception
   D Sexual behaviour
   E Fear

8. Tolerance occurs with:
   A Lithium
   B Barbiturates
   C Heroin
   D Morphia
   E Cocaine

9. The following are personality inventories:
   A Cattell's 16 PF
   B Stanford-Binet test
   C The mandala
   D MMPI
   E Psychoanalytic theory

10. **Factors influencing the rate of conduction of an axon include:**
   A Placebo reactivity
   B Length
   C Degree of neurasthenia
   D Diameter
   E Whether it is myelinated

11. **The following drugs have a half-life exceeding twelve hours:**
   A Chlorpromazine
   B Subcutaneous atropine
   C Amitriptyline
   D Chlordiazepoxide
   E Lithium carbonate

12. **Repression:**
   A Refers to the blocking of an anxiety-producing impulse from awareness
   B Occurs only in childhood
   C Was viewed by Freud as the underlying process upon which the other defence mechanisms are built:
   D Can account for some cases of amnesia
   E If completely successful, results in a total forgetting

13. **The following statements are true of the biosynthesis of noradrenaline from tyrosine:**
   A Dopamine beta hydroxylase is required
   B Phenylalanine is an intermediary
   C Dopamine is formed by the addition of a hydroxyl group to DOPA
   D Tryptophan is an intermediary
   E Noradrenaline is formed by the addition of a hydroxyl group to dopamine

14. **The Wechsler Adult Intelligence Scale:**
   A Is based on free association
   B Tests vocabulary
   C Uses block design tests
   D Is a projective test
   E Tests arithmetical ability

15. **Recognized causes of mental subnormality include:**
A Autosomal trisomies
B Bilateral ECT
C XYY condition
D Deficiency of cystathionine synthetase
E Chromosome deletions

16. **Delusional perception:**
A Is a type of secondary delusion
B Is pathognomic of schizophrenia if organic brain disease can be excluded
C Arises secondary to auditory hallucinations
D Is preceded by a delusional mood in a significant percentage of cases
E Denotes a delusion arising in response to a normal perception

17. **Drug dependence of the morphine type is characterized by:**
A A tendency to reduce the dose
B A relapsing course
C Physical dependence
D Auditory hallucinations
E An abstinence syndrome

18. **Classical conditioning:**
A Was originated by B. F. Skinner
B Uses the concept of undoing
C Was described by Pavlov
D Uses repression
E Is the formation of an association between a conditioned stimulus and a response

19. **Passivity experiences:**
A Occur in schizophrenia
B Are characteristic of obsessional neurosis
C Are listed by Schneider as First Rank Symptoms
D Are evidence against schizophrenia
E Respond rapidly to client-centred psychotherapy

20. Recognized functions of the reticular activating system include control of:
    A Sleep
    B Fine motor skills
    C Arousal
    D The histamine reaction
    E Vigilance

21. The following disorders are transmitted by a single dominant gene:
    A Tuberous sclerosis
    B Phenylketonuria
    C Huntington's Chorea
    D Wilson's disease
    E Down's syndrome (mongolism)

22. Systematic desensitization:
    A Is the same as 'flooding'
    B Is used in the treatment of phobias
    C Involves a hierarchy of feared situations
    D Is a recognized treatment for schizophrenia
    E Is used in conjunction with reciprocal inhibition

23. Characteristic features of atropine poisoning include:
    A Symptoms due to parasympathetic receptor blockade
    B Constricted pupils
    C Bradycardia
    D Visual hallucinations
    E Dryness of the mouth

24. Schizophrenic disorder of thought form includes:
    A Delusions of guilt
    B Overinclusive thinking
    C Impairment of abstract thinking
    D Interpenetration of themes
    E Tactile hallucinations

25. **Transference is:**
    A A defence mechanism of the ego
    B Behaviour by patient towards therapist as if the therapist was an important person from the patient's childhood
    C Based on unconscious mechanisms
    D The process of changing one's therapist
    E The basis of operant conditioning

26. **The following statements are true of electroencephalography:**
    A Alpha waves are predominant from birth
    B Barbiturates slow the rate
    C Dementia is associated with slow activity
    D Theta waves are from 14 to 30 cycles/sec.
    E Diazepam causes fast activity

27. **Extinction refers to:**
    A Loss of transference
    B Loss of an unreinforced behaviour
    C Loss of a conditioned response
    D Termination of behaviour therapy
    E Loss of libido by the therapist

28. **Characteristic features of REM sleep include:**
    A Low voltage EEG waves at 4–10 cycles/sec.
    B Immobility of the eyeballs
    C Dreaming
    D Increase in skeletal muscle tone
    E Cyanosis

29. **The following statements concerning sex chromosomal aberrations are correct:**
    A The incidence in mental hospitals is higher than in the general population
    B XYY condition has an extra Barr body
    C In the multiple X conditions, the more X's, the greater the likelihood of mental subnormality
    D XO is characteristically associated with profound mental subnormality
    E XYY are infertile

30. **The following are true of schizophrenia:**
   A First admission rates are higher for the age 65 years than for the age 25 years
   B Expectation of schizophrenia in a sibling of a schizophrenic is less than 20%
   C Monozygous twin concordance rates, when pooled, are over 20%
   D Monozygous twin concordance rates are typically less than dizygous twin concordance rates
   E Children of a schizophrenic have a lifetime expectation of schizophrenia of less than 3%

31. **Amnestic syndrome is a recognized feature of:**
   A Bilateral hippocampal damage
   B Thiamine deficiency
   C Schizophrenia
   D Bilateral temporal lobectomy
   E Cerebral anoxia

32. **Free association:**
   A Is a result of the Mental Health Act (1959)
   B Is one of the foundations of the psychoanalytic method
   C Is facilitated by repression
   D Has the purpose of bringing to awareness the thoughts and feelings of which the patient is unaware
   E Can occur only if the patient has insight

33. **A secondary delusion:**
   A Occurs in depressive illnesses
   B Is pathognomic of schizophrenia
   C Is usually true
   D Occurs as the result of a hallucination
   E Occurs in paranoid psychoses

34. **The following statements are true of the middle cerebral artery:**
   - A Its two branches are formed by the bifurcation of the basilar artery
   - B The most characteristic symptom of occlusion is contralateral homonymous hemianopsia
   - C Its branches supply portions of the precentral gyrus
   - D It supplies areas responsible for the motor formulation of speech
   - E Contralateral hemiplegia is a recognized complication of occlusion

35. **Recognized features of delirium tremens include:**
   - A Hypokalaemia
   - B Hypomagnesaemia
   - C Excessive sweating
   - D Drowsiness
   - E Hunger

36. **Operant conditioning:**
   - A Was introduced by B. F. Skinner
   - B Refers to increasing the probability of a response by following the response with reinforcement
   - C Can be used for shaping behaviour
   - D Includes the use of secondary reinforcement
   - E Includes the use of tokens

37. **Significant evidence supporting a genetic component to schizophrenia has been provided by:**
   - A The difference between monozygous and dizygous concordance rates in twin studies
   - B The incidence of schizophrenia in the adopted-out children of schizophrenic mothers
   - C Inter-rater reliability studies in the diagnosis of schizophrenia
   - D Individual case reports
   - E Chromosome counts

38. **The following are concepts from ethology:**
A Neuroticism
B Innate releasing mechanism
C Introversion/extroversion
D Imprinting
E Action-specific energy

39. **Korsakoff's psychosis is significantly associated with pathological lesions in the:**
A Mammillary bodies
B Thymus
C Middle cerebral artery
D Thalamus
E Periaqueductal grey matter

40. **Reliability of a research tool:**
A Is a measure of its validity
B Is a measure of the fit of its construct to an acceptable theory
C Is a measure of its ability to obtain consistent results
D Is measured by administering it several times in the same circumstances to similar people.
E Is a measure of its ability to predict an eventuality

41. **Mesial temporal (Ammon's horn) sclerosis is a recognized complication of:**
A Birth injury
B Micropsia
C Coprophagia
D Infantile convulsions
E Bilateral temporal lobectomy

42. The following statements concerning the sympathetic nervous system are correct:
A Adrenaline relaxes bronchii by its action on alpha receptors
B Alpha receptors are blocked by phentolamine
C Beta receptors are stimulated by propanalol
D Adrenaline increases the heart rate by its action on beta receptors
E Adrenaline dilates pupils by its action on beta receptors

43. Double blind trials are recognized as:
A An effective means of comparing two active drugs
B An effective means of comparing an active drugand a placebo
C Including a design in which the judge is not aware of which patient received the drug being tested
D An effective means of comparing the efficacy of individual and group psychotherapy
E Including a design in which the patient is not aware of which patient received the treatment being tested

44. Characteristic features of non-dominant parietal lobe damage include:
A Diplopia
B Confabulation
C Spatial agnosia
D Anosognosia for hemiplegia, if present
E Dressing apraxia

45. Displacement activity, in ethology:
A Is the displacement of surplus aroused energy when the normal discharge is blocked
B Was described by Tinbergen
C Is characteristically associated with supra-normal sign stimuli
D Is demonstrated in birds by pecking grass instead of fighting when confronted by a larger opponent
E Occurs characteristically during a critical period

46. The following structures form part of the limbic system:
  A Fornix
  B Amygdala
  C Vermis of the cerebellum
  D Hippocampus
  E Septal nuclei

47. Tests of schizophrenic thought disorder include the:
  A WAIS
  B Guthrie test
  C Bannister and Fransella test
  D Repertory Grid
  E Object classification and sorting tests

48. In the normal distribution:
  A Greater than 95% of the distribution lies within three standard deviations below the mean and three standard deviations above the mean
  B Less than 50% of the population are within one standard deviation below the mean and one standard deviation above the mean
  C The curve is asymmetric
  D The mean and median fall at the same point
  E The mode and mean fall at the same point

49. The following statements concerning thiamine deficiency are correct:
  A It results in cerebral accumulation of pyruvate
  B It causes a reduction in transketolase activity
  C It results in lesions in the mammillary bodies
  D It is significantly associated with the use of marihuana
  E It is significantly associated with alcoholism

50. Recognized techniques of behaviour therapy include:
  A Desensitization
  B Flooding
  C Reciprocal inhibition
  D Somatic passivity
  E Imprinting

51. **Factors having a recognized influence on intelligence test performance include:**
A Motivation
B Anxiety
C Fatigue
D Heredity
E Age

52. **Characteristic features of Gerstmann's syndrome include:**
A Ophthalmoplegia
B Finger agnosia
C Acalculia
D Agraphia
E Ataxia

53. **Projection:**
A Is an ego defence mechanism
B Typically does not occur in normal people
C Is another name for repression
D Typically occurs in paranoid states
E Is an unconscious process which protects against anxiety

54. **Imprinting:**
A Is strengthened by punishment
B Is the explanation of behaviour changes in psychotherapy
C Characteristically occurs during a critical period
D Is found only in birds
E Has been demonstrated by Lorenz

55. **Characteristic features of the Kluver–Bucy syndrome include:**
A Visual agnosia
B Korsakoff's psychosis
C Lack of fear
D Hypersexuality
E Oral exploration

56. Psychological tests of organic brain disease include:
- A MMPI
- B New word learning tests
- C Rorschach
- D Personality inventories
- E Memory-for-designs tests

57. Parasympathetic actions characteristically include:
- A Dilatation of the pupil
- B Decrease in heart rate
- C Decrease in salivation
- D Bronchial constriction
- E Decrease in peristalsis

58. Incidence refers to:
- A The number of new cases emerging in a designated period and population
- B The point prevalence of an illness
- C The period prevalence of an illness
- D The readmission rate
- E The number of beds occupied in a designated population

59. The following disorders are typically transmitted by an X-linked gene:
- A Homocystinuria
- B Glucose-6-phosphate dehydrogenase deficiency
- C Hunter's syndrome (gargoylism)
- D Galactosaemia
- E Niemann–Pick disease

60. For an effective comparison of two treatments, the following statements are correct:

A Matching in pairs is a satisfactory way of assignment of patients to treatment groups

B Random assignment is the only safe way of assignment to treatment groups

C Double blind procedures are absolutely essential

D Treatment outcome should be evaluated by independent measures

E Matching of total groups before treatment allows for different amounts of kind of dropouts

Paper 2

1. Mirror gazing is a recognized feature of:
   A Anorexia nervosa
   B Delirium tremens
   C Hebephrenic schizophrenia
   D Alzheimer's disease
   E Manic-depressive psychosis

2. The cerebellum contains the following:
   A Dentate nucleus
   B Substantia nigra
   C Vermis
   D Hippocampus
   E Globus pallidus

3. Anterior-pituitary function is regulated by:
   A The nigro-striatal pathway
   B Hypothalamic control
   C CNS control
   D Negative-feedback control
   E Environmental stimuli

4. Chlormethiazole:
   A Is a hypnotic
   B is epileptogenic
   C Has muscle-relaxing properties
   D Is effective in the treatment of alcohol withdrawal
   E Is structurally related to thiamine

5. **Extinction:**
   - A Includes a gradual loss of the conditioned response
   - B Occurs in operant conditioning
   - C Refers to the ending of a psychotherapeutic relationship
   - D Occurs in classical conditioning when the unconditioned stimulus is omitted repeatedly
   - E Results from repetition of the conditioned stimulus without reinforcement

6. **The following statements concerning vitamin B12 deficiency are correct:**
   - A Specific treatment is intramuscular replacement therapy
   - B The tongue is usually furred
   - C There is a favourable response to a combination of nicotinic acid and tryptophan
   - D Ankle jerks are decreased or absent
   - E Achlorhydria is often present

7. **Characteristic symptoms of frontal lobe syndrome include:**
   - A Organic hallucinosis
   - B Indifference to the feelings of others
   - C A general lack of drive
   - D Lack of foresight
   - E Loss of memory

8. **Characteristic symptoms of Korsakoff's psychosis include:**
   - A Confabulation
   - B Disorientation for time
   - C Catatonia
   - D Narcolepsy
   - E Echolalia

9. **Agoraphobia:**
   - A Is a characteristic feature of schizophrenia
   - B Is associated with promiscuity in the majority of cases
   - C Is a fear of going into open spaces
   - D Is commoner in females
   - E Is a characteristic feature of hypomania

10. **The following statements concerning drugs and the Central Nervous System are correct:**
   - A Drugs which are highly bound to plasma albumin tend to enter the brain more quickly than poorly bound drugs
   - B In cerebrospinal fluid, the majority of drug present is bound to protein
   - C Passage of a drug across the blood–brain barrier is more rapid with the non-ionized form of the drug than with the ionized form
   - D Lipid solubility of the non-ionized form of a drug is a more important factor in governing the rate of diffusion than the lipid solubility of the ionized form of the drug
   - E Brain tissue does not bind drugs

11. **Appropriate investigations for suspected thiamine deficiency include:**
   - A Blood transketolase activity
   - B Pyruvate tolerance test
   - C Oxygen-15 brain studies
   - D Serum lithium estimation
   - E Isotope encephalography

12. **Plethysmography is a recognized technique for:**
   - A The treatment of schizophrenia
   - B Assessing physical correlates of anxiety in the experimental situation
   - C Measuring changes in penile volume
   - D The measurement of blood flow for experimental purposes
   - E The emergency treatment of cat-scratch disease

13. **Characteristic features of opiate withdrawal include:**
   - A Mydriasis
   - B Piloerection
   - C Constipation
   - D Hunger
   - E Rhinorrhoea

14. **Recognized features of Personal Construct Theory include:**
    A Use of the paired-associate learning test
    B The organization of bipolar concepts
    C Use of the repertory grid technique
    D Overinclusiveness estimation
    E The measurement of concreteness

15. **According to Lorenz, characteristics in which human societies differ from wolf packs include:**
    A Hypertrophy of drive for food intake
    B Hypertrophy of drive for mating
    C Individuals with behavioural deficiencies are more socially handicapped
    D Increase in social inhibitions
    E Reduction in social drives

16. **A delusion is a belief which:**
    A Is not true to fact
    B Cannot be corrected by an appeal to the reason of the person entertaining it
    C Is out of harmony with the individual's education and surroundings
    D Is typically accompanied by insight
    E Invariably occurs secondary to a hallucination

17. **The following groups have a higher prevalence of EEG abnormalities than does the general population:**
    A Psychopaths
    B Airline pilots
    C Schizophrenics
    D Epileptics
    E Neurotics

18. **The following are commoner in the prison population of UK than in the general population:**
    A Females
    B Temporal lobe EEG abnormalities
    C Psychopathic personality disorder
    D Schizophrenia
    E History of juvenile delinquency

19. **Temporal lobe epilepsy is significantly associated with:**
   - A Hypnosis
   - B Schizophreniform psychosis
   - C Deja vu phenomena
   - D Cerebral tumour
   - E Thiamine deficiency

20. **Obsessive compulsive thoughts:**
   - A Are effectively treated with phenothiazines
   - B Are recognized by the patient as his own
   - C Are ego-syntonic
   - D Are typically described by the patient as enjoyable
   - E Are usually in a foreign language

21. **Dopamine is found in the:**
   - A Caudate nucleus
   - B Cerebral cortex
   - C Substantia nigra
   - D Cerebellar neuroglia
   - E Amygdala

22. **Chromosomes:**
   - A Are of dominant or recessive types
   - B Are normal in Mongolism (Down's syndrome)
   - C Consist fundamentally of deoxyribonucleic acid (DNA)
   - D Split longitudinally in meiosis
   - E Number 48 in the normal human somatic cells, excluding the gametes

23. **Characteristics of autosomal recessive inheritance include:**
   - A The parents are more commonly affected than they are in dominant inheritance
   - B A proportion of one in four siblings of patients with recessive forms of mental defect are expected to be affected
   - C A proportion of one in four siblings of patients with recessive forms of mental defect are expected to be symptomless carriers
   - D An increased incidence of parental consanguinity
   - E Late age of onset of manifestation in phenotype

24. **The following concepts are typically associated with the name Piaget:**
    - A Sensorimotor period
    - B Period of concrete operations
    - C Preoperational phase
    - D Neuroticism
    - E Maternal deprivation

25. **The following names are typically associated with the concept of mothering:**
    - A Milgram
    - B Festinger
    - C Rorschach
    - D Harlow
    - E Bowlby

26. **Sheldon's classification of body-typing includes the following components:**
    - A Endomorphic
    - B Mesomorphic
    - C Acromegalic
    - D Pyknic
    - E Choleric

27. **Recognized causes of cerebral atrophy include:**
    - A Paranoia
    - B General paresis of the insane
    - C Delirium
    - D Phobic-anxiety depersonalization syndrome
    - E Huntington's chorea

28. **Characteristic features of petit mal epilepsy include:**
    - A 3 per second spike and wave on EEG
    - B Initial onset in adult life
    - C Progression to grand mal epilepsy
    - D Deja vu experiences
    - E Progression to cerebral atrophy

29. **The phenomena of alcoholic hallucinosis:**
   A Consist of pseudo-hallucinations
   B Include auditory hallucinations only if there is a family history of schizophrenia
   C Usually occur at the beginning of a drinking bout
   D Are significantly associated with delirium tremens
   E Are typically described by the patient as enjoyable

30. **Recognized clinical tests of the second cranial nerve include:**
   A Pupillary light reflex
   B Visual field determination
   C Visual acuity
   D Queckenstedt test
   E Tests for Romberg's sign

31. **Reflexes typically associated with directing the eyes to an object close at hand include:**
   A Delayed ankle jerks
   B Convergence
   C Accommodation
   D Ciliospinal reflex
   E Pupillary constriction

32. **Recognized signs of lithium intoxication include:**
   A Hunger
   B Coarse tremor
   C Slurred speech
   D Diarrhoea
   E Ataxia

33. **Recognized features of eighth cranial nerve disorder include:**
   A Hearing loss
   B Tinnitus
   C The Weber test lateralizes to the normal ear
   D Bone conduction is better than air conduction
   E A threshold deficit in the reception of tones in the higher frequencies

34. **Workers whose contributions have typically involved animal experimentation include:**
 A Seligman
 B Harlow
 C Clifford Beers
 D Brady
 E R. D. Laing

35. **Recognized side effects of phenytoin include:**
 A Gum hyperplasia
 B Ataxia
 C Hirsutism
 D Epileptic fits
 E Folate depletion

36. **Recognized causes of nystagmus include:**
 A Anosmia
 B Degeneration of the substantia nigra
 C Irritation of the eighth cranial nerve
 D Damage to the vestibular nuclei
 E Acute alcohol intoxication

37. **The following statements concerning releasers which inhibit aggressive behaviour are correct:**
 A An example is submissive posturing
 B They are typically effective in encounters with animals of the same species
 C They typically consist of presentation of a specific vulnerable part of the body
 D They are commoner in herbivores than in carnivores
 E They are characteristically more effective in the inhibition of impersonal aggression such as bombing than in the inhibition of aggression during hand to hand combat

38. Eyelid conditioning experiments typically show that:
    A Patients with animal phobias have rapid conditioning
    B REM sleep deprivation is a factor in the aetiology of schizophrenia
    C Agoraphobics tend to condition slowly
    D Patients with social phobias show no particular conditioning characteristics
    E Patients with animal phobias have slow extinction

39. Recognized features of the inheritance of Huntington's chorea include:
    A The involvement of more than one locus
    B A single major gene
    C Transmission as an autosomal dominant
    D Gene penetrance over 90%
    E Y-linked recessive mutation in the female

40. The following are projective tests:
    A Rod and frame test
    B Body sway suggestibility
    C Pursuit rotor
    D Dark adaptation
    E Thematic Apperception Test

41. Recognized side effects of phenothiazines include:
    A Photosensitive dermatitis
    B Akathisia
    C Jaundice
    D Retinitis pigmentosa
    E Weight gain

42. Recognized functions of the trigeminal nerve include:
    A Sensation from the skin of the face
    B Innervation of the skeletal musculature of the tongue
    C Innervation of cardiac muscle
    D Sensation from mucous membranes of the nasal chamber
    E Innervation of the lateral rectus muscle

43. **Recognized features of phenylketonuria include:**
- A An increased incidence in Jews
- B Inheritance as an autosomal recessive trait
- C Mental subnormality
- D Delay in onset of harmful effects until after commencement of the reproductive period
- E Increased incidence of cousin marriages in the parents

44. **Schneiderian First Rank symptoms of schizophrenia include:**
- A Poor empathy
- B Autism
- C Ambivalence
- D Somatic passivity
- E Delusional perception

45. **Structures involved in the corneal reflex include:**
- A Trigeminal nerve
- B Facial nerve
- C Orbicularis oculi muscle
- D Oculomotor nerve
- E Accessory nerve

46. **The following statements concerning cluster analysis are correct:**
- A It is a statistical technique for sorting people into groups
- B It assumes a continuous distribution of the variables being assessed
- C It is the same as factor analysis
- D It is the basis of intelligence testing
- E It was invented by Barbara Wootton

47. **The personality constellation of high extroversion plus high neuroticism is significantly associated with:**
- A Depression
- B Accident proneness
- C Likelihood of becoming an unmarried mother
- D Obsessionality
- E Psychopathic behaviour

48. **Factor analysis typically involves the use of:**
- A Intercorrelations
- B A matrix
- C Rotation of axes
- D Observer rating scales
- E Evoked potentials

49. **Drugs characteristically causing tachycardia include:**
- A Atropine
- B Propanalol
- C Acetylcholine
- D Marihuana
- E Adrenaline

50. **Branches of the vagus nerve include:**
- A Cochlear
- B Recurrent laryngeal
- C Cardiac
- D Olivocerebellar
- E Superior laryngeal

51. **The properties of a normal (Gaussian) curve can be described completely by stating:**
- A Mean and standard deviation
- B Mode and mean
- C Median and mean
- D Median, mode and mean
- E Median and standard deviation

52. **Hallucinations are significantly associated with:**
- A Mongolism (Down's syndrome)
- B Sensory deprivation
- C Hypnosis
- D Psychotic depression
- E Sociopathic personality traits

53. **Recognized consequences of carotid sinus stimulation include:**
   A Syncope
   B Slowing of the heart rate
   C Increase in blood pressure
   D Vasodilation of peripheral blood vessels
   E Elevation of intracranial pressure

54. **Typical uses of the product-moment correlation formula include:**
   A Calculation of the correlation coefficient
   B Calculations of comparisons across different types of measures
   C Factor analysis
   D Calculation of standard deviation
   E Calculation of mode

55. **Recognized features of Tuberous Sclerosis (Epiloia) include:**
   A Sex-linked inheritance
   B Epilepsy
   C Dominant inheritance
   D Mental subnormality
   E Variable expressivity with respect to intelligence

56. **The following statements are correct:**
   A Values of the correlation coefficient required for significance at the 5% level are independent of sample size
   B A high correlation implies direct causation
   C A correlation of $r = 0.50$ is indicative of only 25% of common elements shared by x and y
   D A correlation of $r = 0.30$ indicates only 9% of common elements between x and y
   E The null hypothesis refers to the significance of statistical data

57. **Recognized side-effects of propanolol include:**
  - A Bronchospasm
  - B Congestive heart failure
  - C Retinal degeneration
  - D Tachycardia
  - E Hyperglycaemia

58. **Characteristic features of acute salicylate poisoning include:**
  - A Coma
  - B Vomiting
  - C Tinnitus
  - D Respiratory acidosis
  - E Sweating

59. **Nocturnal eneuresis with daytime control at the age of five years:**
  - A Is significantly associated with ectopic ureter
  - B Is appropriately investigated by a voiding cystogram
  - C Is best treated with amphetamines
  - D Is a recognized indication for circumcision
  - E Is characteristically associated with severe emotional disturbance

60. **Characteristic features of schizophrenia include:**
  - A Memory impairment
  - B Auditory hallucination in clear consciousness
  - C Disturbance of thought processes
  - D Feelings of panic in buses and shops
  - E A feeling of being under the influence of an external force

Paper 3

1. Coefficients for measuring the covariability between a pair of concomitant variables include:
   A Latin square
   B Mode
   C Product moment correlation
   D Rank correlation coefficient
   E Reliability coefficient

2. Releasing schema for human parental care responses include:
   A Large eyes
   B Clumsy movements
   C Low-lying eyes
   D Long extremities
   E Hollow cheek region

3. Peripheral neuro-endocrine mechanisms involved in anxiety states:
   A Are typically under voluntary control
   B Were described by the James–Lange theory
   C Were described by Cannon's hypothesis
   D Include discharge of the sympathetic autonomic nervous system
   E Include discharge of the nigro-striatal pathways

4. **The Papez circuit includes:**
   A Vagus nerve
   B Mammillothalamic tract
   C Hippocampus
   D Fornix
   E Optic radiation

5. **Children with IQ's below fifty (50):**
   A Tend to come from families where the parental IQ is very low
   B Inherit a Mendelian autosomal dominant condition in the majority of cases
   C Are able eventually to earn their own living in the majority of cases
   D Are the result of regression towards the mean
   E Have a single gene disorder in the majority of cases

6. **Recognized causes of anosmia include:**
   A Meningitis
   B Fracture of the ethmoid bone
   C Cerebellar astrocytoma
   D Congenital absence of the corpus callosum
   E The common cold

7. **Recognized methods of data collection include:**
   A Direct observation
   B Extrapolation
   C Interviewing
   D Abstraction from published statistics
   E Interpolation

8. **In the experimental situation, increase in forearm blood-flow is a recognized feature of:**
   A Severe chronic anxiety
   B Medication with diazepam
   C Personality disorder
   D Depersonalization
   E Subjects with low self-ratings of anxiety

9. **The following statements concerning action-specific arousal modality and behavioural motivation are correct:**
   - A The stimulus threshold sinks in the absence of con-specific surroundings
   - B The stimulus threshold sinks during periods without response
   - C The stimulus threshold rises following abreaction of the drive concerned
   - D Endogenous accumulation of response-specific behavioural motivation occurs
   - E Members of expeditions are typically unmoved by minor irritations

10. **Lesions in the following areas typically result in aphasia:**
   - A The cerebellum
   - B Broca's area of the dominant hemisphere
   - C The posterior part of the superior temporal gyrus of the dominant hemisphere
   - D The posterior part of the temporal lobe of the non-dominant hemisphere
   - E The occipital lobe of the non-dominant hemisphere

11. **Recognized features of high extroversion include:**
   - A The finding that stimulant drugs have a normalizing effect on objective behaviour tests
   - B Stimulus hunger
   - C Lower pain threshold
   - D Increased susceptibility to the adverse effects of sensory deprivation
   - E Impairment in utilizing learned patterns of behaviour

12. **Basal ganglia include:**
   - A Caudate nucleus
   - B Dentate nucleus
   - C Putamen
   - D Globus pallidus
   - E Lentiform nucleus

13. The following statements concerning Klinefelter's syndrome are correct:
   A It is commoner in females
   B It is invariably associated with sterility
   C It is commoner in old age
   D It occurs typically as an X-linked recessive inheritance
   E A proportion of patients are chromatin-positive

14. Recognized techniques for describing the relationship between two variables include:
   A Scattergram
   B Harmonic mean
   C Regression lines
   D Use of percentiles
   E Correlation coefficient

15. Hormones of the anterior lobe of the pituitary (adenohypophysis) include:
   A Growth hormone
   B ACTH
   C Oxytocin
   D Luteinizing hormone
   E Vasopressin

16. The following are recognized experiences of a normal fully-conscious person:
   A Delusional perception
   B Deja vu
   C Denial
   D Projection
   E Voices repeating one's thoughts aloud

17. **The following statements concerning tardive dyskinesia are correct:**
   - A It is significantly associated with the treatment of chronic schizophrenia
   - B It is effectively treated by intra-muscular benztropine
   - C It occurs predominantly in young females
   - D Benhexol is an effective prophylactic
   - E Reducing the dose of a phenothiazine is a recognized precipitant

18. **The following statements concerning the XYY syndrome are correct:**
   - A It is most common in tall lesbian females
   - B It is characteristically associated with stunted growth in the male
   - C A pathognomic feature is webbing of the neck
   - D The basic pathological lesion is in the ovaries
   - E There is a significant association with criminality

19. **Characteristics of a perfect positive correlation include:**
   - A An increase in one variable is associated with an increase in the other
   - B A change in one variable is matched by a change of equal degree in the other variable
   - C All the points of the scattergraph lie on the line of best fit
   - D A Pearson product-moment coefficient of correlation of value zero (0)
   - E Absence of spurious correlation

20. **Cattell's sixteen primary factors include:**
   - A Intelligence
   - B MMPI factor
   - C Conservatism
   - D Neuroticism
   - E Extroversion

21. **In the development of domesticated races of animals the following changes from ancestral forms occur in the majority of cases:**
    - A Reduction in selectivity of innate releasing schema
    - B Expansion of sexual releasing mechanisms
    - C Increase in quality of parental care
    - D Increase in promiscuity
    - E Retardation of locomotor organs

22. **Recognized features of Turner's syndrome include:**
    - A The triple-X constitution (XXX)
    - B Lack of development of secondary sexual characteristics
    - C Shortness of stature
    - D Chromatin-negative smears
    - E A male incidence of red-green colour blindness

23. **Eysenck and the British school have derived the following personality factors:**
    - A Extroversion–introversion
    - B Cerebrotonia
    - C Dysplasia
    - D Psychoticism
    - E Neuroticism

24. **Tests which characteristically measure the statistical significance include:**
    - A Chi-squared
    - B Those which test the null hypothesis
    - C t-test
    - D Probability (p) tests
    - E Validity tests

25. **The pupillary light reflex pathway includes:**
    - A Superior colliculus
    - B Edinger–Westphal nucleus
    - C Cranial nerve III
    - D Dentate gyrus
    - E Fimbria

26. **Hypertensive reactions are a recognized complication of the interaction of Monoamine Oxidase Inhibitors with:**
    A Tyramine
    B Cough mixtures
    C Cheese
    D Methylamphetamine
    E Phenylpropanolamine

27. **Grandiose delusions are recognized symptoms of:**
    A Anorexia nervosa
    B Mania
    C General paresis of the insane
    D Depressive psychosis
    E Schizophrenia

28. **Recognized behaviour therapy treatments for phobias include:**
    A Desensitization
    B Imprinting
    C Token economies
    D Modelling
    E Flooding

29. **Recognized side-effects of benzhexol include:**
    A Blurred vision
    B Dry mouth
    C Toxic psychosis
    D Parkinsonism
    E Visual hallucinations

30. **Concrete thinking is a recognized symptom of:**
    A Neurosis
    B Schizophrenia
    C Coarse brain disease
    D Mild mental subnormality
    E Personality disorder

31. **The following statements concerning the Yerkes–Dodson law are correct:**
   - A The optimum level of aversive stimulation in the control of learning is at some moderate intensity, lower and higher values being less effective
   - B It produces a straight line on a normal scale graph
   - C The optimum level of motivation for learning decreases with increasing task difficulty
   - D It is a generalization that serves as a model for the relationship between affective intensity and adaptive behaviour
   - E There is a constant positive correlation between arousal and performance

32. **The following statements concerning the Barr body are correct:**
   - A It consists mainly of DNA
   - B If one Barr body is present, the cell can be assumed to contain one X chromosome and one Y chromosome
   - C It is found in the cell nucleus
   - D The buccal smear test is of value only in cats
   - E It enables the detection of individuals in whom the nuclear sex is at variance with the phenotypical sex

33. **Behaviour therapy techniques include the use of:**
   - A Negative practice
   - B Apomorphine
   - C Extinction
   - D Shaping
   - E Free association

34. **Euphoria is a recognized symptom of:**
   - A Disseminated sclerosis
   - B Mania
   - C General paresis
   - D Frontal lobe lesions
   - E Hebephrenic schizophrenia

35. **Recognized explanations of the occurrence of a hereditary illness when parents are both clinically normal include:**
    A Autosomal recessive inheritance
    B Polygenic inheritance
    C The occurrence of a fresh mutation
    D Variability in the manifestation of the gene
    E Parental consanguity

36. **The following statements concerning the Minnesota Multiphasic Personality Inventory are correct:**
    A The selection of scales is based on factor analysis
    B It includes a scale for 'endomorphy'
    C It includes a scale for 'hypochondriasis'
    D It consists of standard rating scales compiled by interviewers personally acquainted with the patient
    E It includes a scale for 'paranoia'

37. **The ciliary muscle of the eye responds to the following drugs:**
    A Parasympathomimetics
    B Parasympatholytics
    C sympathomimetics
    D Sympatholytics
    E Atropine

38. **The Monoamine Theory of Affective Disturbances relies on the following evidence:**
    A Chemical substances which cause depression decrease the amount of monoamines available at synapses
    B Physical treatments that are effective in depression tend to increase the amount of monoamines available to central receptors
    C In spontaneously arising depression, there is evidence of a diminution in monoamine synthesis
    D Only a minority of patients treated with Monoamine Oxidase Inhibitors develop acute hypertension
    E When hypertension does occur, it is relieved by the injection of phentolamine

39. **Characteristic symptoms of hypomania include:**
A Confabulation
B Lack of consideration for others
C Deja vu experiences
D Pressure of speech
E Overactivity

40. **Cushing's syndrome is typically associated with:**
A Excessive production of glucocorticoids by the adrenal cortex
B Adrenocortical hyperplasia
C Depression
D Anorexia nervosa
E Pituitary tumour

41. **Thiamine deficiency is a recognized cause of:**
A Alcoholic hallucinosis
B Wernicke's encephalopathy
C Polyneuritis
D Pellagra
E Alcoholic tremulousness

42. **Structures involved in the perception of pain include:**
A Ventral roots of the spinal nerves
B Lateral spino-thalamic tract
C Parietal cortex
D Thalamus
E Vermis of the cerebellum

43. **Akathisia:**
A Is typically associated with malingering
B Is appropriately treated with diazepam
C Is typically enjoyable to the patient
D Is a recognized side-effect of phenothiazines
E Is a recognized side-effect of butyrophenones

44. **Disorientation for time is a characteristic symptom of:**
A Korsakoff's psychosis
B Acute schizophrenia
C Hypomania
D Dementia
E Delirium

45. **Recognized consequences of injury to an individual peripheral nerve include:**
A Spastic paralysis
B Loss of all forms of sensation except proprioception
C Muscular weakness
D Muscular atrophy
E Subacute combined degeneration of the spinal cord

46. **Characteristic symptoms of endogenous (psychotic) depression include:**
A Apathy
B Pessimism
C Guilt
D Suicidal ideas
E Visual hallucinations of small objects

47. **The following statements are true of acetylcholine in the nervous system:**
A It is the chemical transmitter of the parasympathetic nervous system
B It is absent from the brain
C Some receptors are blocked by atropine
D Some receptors are blocked by curare
E It stimulates beta receptors in the sympathetic nervous system

48. **The following statements concerning the rate of uptake of drugs from the blood into the brain are correct:**
A Dopamine is taken up more rapidly than levodopa
B Serotonin is taken up more rapidly than tryptophan
C Thiopentone is taken up more rapidly than barbitone
D Physostigmine is taken up more rapidly than neostigmine
E Lithium ions are taken up more rapidly than dopamine

49. **Recognized consequences of tabes dorsalis include:**
    - A Parasthesias
    - B Attacks of sharp pain
    - C Diminished sensitivity to painful stimuli
    - D A negative Romberg sign
    - E Increased ankle jerks

50. **Schneiderian first rank symptoms of schizophrenia include:**
    - A Made impulses
    - B Visual hallucinations
    - C Paranoid delusions
    - D Incongruity of effect
    - E Loosening of associations

51. **Phobia:**
    - A Is commoner in men than in women
    - B Responds rapidly to analytically orientated group psychotherapy
    - C Cannot be reasoned away
    - D Leads to avoidance of the feared situation
    - E Is treated successfully by systematic desensitization

52. **Recognized consequences of syringomelia include:**
    - A Loss of proprioception
    - B Interruption of the lateral spinothalamic fibres which cross from one side to the other
    - C Loss of simple touch sensibility
    - D Loss of pain sensibility
    - E Loss of temperature sensibility

53. **Cells of the neuroglia include:**
    - A Astrocytes
    - B Oligodendrocytes
    - C Microglia
    - D Neurones
    - E Purkinje cells

54. The following writers are known for their work on the effects of electroconvulsive therapy:
   A Pinel
   B Ottoson
   C Tinbergen
   D D'Elia
   E Pasteur

55. Hallucinations of touch are significantly associated with:
   A Cocaine psychosis
   B Schizophrenia
   C Obsessional neurosis
   D Fugues
   E Conversion neurosis

56. Recognized features of thiamine deficiency include:
   A Nystagmus
   B Polyneuritis
   C Ataxia
   D Oculomotor disturbances
   E Wernicke's encephalopathy

57. Hallucinations in schizophrenia are recognized to include the following modalities:
   A Auditory
   B Visual
   C Tactile
   D Body shape
   E Olfactory

58. Delusions are a recognized feature of:
   A Delirium tremens
   B Obsessional neurosis
   C Homosexuality
   D Pathological jealousy
   E Hypomania

59. Characteristic features of endogenous depression include:
   A Feelings of passivity
   B Feelings of guilt
   C Early morning waking
   D Grandiose delusions
   E Agoraphobia

60. The following statements regarding alcoholism are correct:
   A It is commoner in males than in females
   B Hallucinations during delirium tremens are characteristically of a visual kind
   C After they have been abstinent for one year, patients are able to resume social drinking
   D It is significantly associated with depression
   E The prognosis is worse in female than in male patients

Paper 4

1. There is a significant correlation between IQ and:
   A EEG evoked potential latency period
   B EEG evoked potential amplitude
   C Parental IQ
   D Foster-parent IQ
   E Sibling IQ

2. The following statements concerning synaptic transmitter substances are correct:
   A Their mode of action includes an increase in post-synaptic membrane permeability
   B They depolarize the post-synaptic cell membrane
   C Excess substance is reabsorbed by the pre-synaptic nerve terminal
   D Excess substance is broken down by enzymes
   E They are responsible for maintaining the resting membrane potential

3. Characteristics of monozygotic (MZ) pairs of twins include:
   A Their origin from splitting of a single zygote
   B Their origin from fertilization of two separate ova
   C The same phenotypic sex
   D An incidence rate of less than 10% of all twins in the general population
   E Higher concordance rates than dizygotic (DZ) pairs

4. **Symptoms due to secondary gain:**
   A Are appropriately treated by succinylcholine apnoea
   B Are appropriately treated by operant conditioning
   C Are appropriately treated by admission to hospital
   D Are perpetuated by reinforcement
   E Typically delay surrender of the sick role

5. **Techniques of multivariate analysis include:**
   A T-groups
   B Self-analysis
   C Psychoanalysis
   D Factor analysis
   E Multiple regression analysis

6. **Vitamin deficiencies are typically associated with:**
   A Alcoholism
   B Senile dementia
   C Obesity
   D Mongolism (Down's syndrome)
   E Agoraphobia

7. **Evidence supporting a genetic component to intelligence includes:**
   A Foster children studies
   B A parent of IQ 80 is likely to have a child of even lower IQ
   C Twin studies
   D Kinship relations
   E A parent of IQ 140 is likely to have a child of even higher IQ

8. **Factors recognized as contributing to disruption of social behaviour patterns include:**
   A Accumulation of action-specific energy
   B The invention of weapons
   C Failure of species-specific inhibition releasers
   D Increasing anonymity of society
   E Misplaced social defence responses

9. **The following statements concerning non-parametric tests are correct:**
   A They need a smaller sample than do parametric tests:
   B They are less sensitive than parametric tests
   C An example is the 't' test
   D They do not make assumptions about the parameters of the population
   E Their power efficiency is lower

10. **Korsakoff's psychosis is typically associated with:**
   A Bradycardia
   B An inability to learn new material
   C Disorientation in time
   D Confabulation
   E Thiamine excess

11. **Factors typically involved in the control of aggression include:**
   A Amygdaloid nucleus
   B Action-specific energy
   C Adrenalin
   D Cerebellum
   E Submissive postures

12. **The beneficial effect of electroconvulsive therapy is recognized as being significantly associated with:**
   A The occurrence of a fit
   B The amperage
   C The psychological set of the anaesthetist
   D The amount of atropine used
   E The symptom pattern of the illness

13. **Hypothyroidism is significantly associated with:**
   A Lithium therapy
   B An increased rate of blood flow through the cerebral cortex
   C Mental lethargy
   D Tardive dyskinesia
   E Depression

14. **Binocular vision is a characteristic of the following:**
A Sticklebacks
B Monkeys
C Mammals which climb trees by means of grasping branches with their extremities
D Marsupials which are grasp-climbers
E Squirrels

15. **Negative practice:**
A Involves massed practice of a learned response
B Is appropriate treatment for tics
C Is appropriate treatment for schizophrenia
D Is appropriate treatment for stammering
E Aims at extinction

16. **Agoraphobics typically:**
A Score low on questionnaire tests of neuroticism
B Are extroverted
C Have a low level of arousal
D Transmit their illness by a sex-linked recessive gene
E Have a specific fear of snakes

17. **Illnesses which characteristically lead to pre-senile dementia include:**
A Alzheimer's disease
B Manic depressive psychosis
C Simple schizophrenia
D Huntington's chorea
E Pick's disease

18. **Structures involved in the direct light reflex include:**
A Optic nerve
B Optic tract
C Ciliary ganglion
D Occipital lobes
E Oculomotor nerve

19. Graphs of frequency distribution include:
    A Histograms
    B Frequency polygon
    C Frequency curve
    D Bar charts
    E Pie charts

20. The personality constellation of high introversion plus high neuroticism is significantly associated with:
    A Anxiety state
    B Hysteria
    C Parachute-jumping
    D Impotence
    E Phobias

21. Characteristic features of Horner's syndrome include:
    A Ataxia
    B Pupillary constriction
    C Sweating on the affected side
    D Ptosis of the eyelid
    E Paralysis of the lower part of the face

22. Chromosomal aberrations include:
    A Inversion
    B Deletion
    C Duplication
    D Translocation
    E Aneuploidy

23. Characteristics of a skewed distribution include:
    A Spurious correlation
    B The mode is always at the peak of the distribution
    C The mode is separated from the mean
    D The mean lies on the side of the longer tail
    E The median always lies on the mode

24. Characteristic results of stimulation of the sympathetic nervous system include:
    A Bradycardia
    B Contraction of the spleen
    C Increased peristalsis
    D Increase of blood pressure
    E Constriction of coronary arteries

25. Nalorphine:
   A Causes dilatation of the pupils in narcotic addicts
   B Is used in the treatment of thiamine deficiency
   C Causes constriction of the pupils in non-narcotic dependent subjects
   D Prevents withdrawal symptoms in morphine addicts
   E Is effective when taken by mouth

26. Characteristics of autosomal dominant inheritance include:
   A Increased incidence of parental consanguinuity
   B An expected incidence of 50% in parents of an affected child
   C An expected incidence of 50% in siblings
   D An expected incidence of 50% in children of an affected parent
   E 'Skipping' a generation

27. Learning theory is significantly associated with the following names:
   A Thorndike
   B Adolf Meyer
   C Hull
   D Watson
   E Festinger

28. Biochemical changes in affective (depressive)psychosis include:
   A Increased serum lithium level in the untreated patient
   B Reduction of cerebral 5-hydroxytryptamine
   C Characteristic increase in free thyroxine in the blood
   D Decreased CSF 5-hydroxyindoles
   E Increase in 'residual sodium'

29. Measures of dispersion (variation) include:
   A Mode
   B Quartile deviation
   C Range
   D Postal questionnaires
   E Standard deviation

30. **Aversion therapy includes the use of:**
A Succinylcholine apnoea
B Electric shocks
C A classical conditioning paradigm
D Massed practice
E Apomorphine

31. **Characteristic features of mongolism (Down's syndrome) include:**
A Trisomy
B An IQ above 50 in the majority of subjects
C Translocation in a minority of subjects
D Increased incidence with increased maternal age
E Chromosome count of 49

32. **Recognized features of the inheritance of hypomania include:**
A Increased incidence of bipolar affective psychosis in relatives
B Increased incidence of hypomania in relatives
C The affected children of affected males are exclusively females
D The illness is twice as common in males as in females
E Pooled monozygous twin concordance rates are typically lower than pooled dizygous twin con-concordance rates

33. **The following statements correctly apply to *both* systematic desensitization and flooding:**
A Both are appropriate treatments for phobias
B Both are appropriate treatments for eneuresis
C Both are appropriate treatments for alcoholism
D Both are based on the principle of reciprocal inhibition
E Both are techniques of behaviour therapy

34. **Recognized consequences of adrenal insufficiency include:**
    - A Sodium retention
    - B Hyperkalaemia
    - C Hypertension
    - D Hypoglycaemia
    - E Pigmentation

35. **Alpha-methyldopa:**
    - A Interferes with the synthesis of noradrenaline at sympathetic nerve endings
    - B Competes with DOPA in a biological pathway
    - C Causes depression in a significant number of patients
    - D Is an intermediary in the normal biological pathway between DOPA and dopamine
    - E Is a proprietary preparation of rauwolfia

36. **Recognized consequences of hemisection of the spinal cord include the following,** *on the side of the lesion:*
    - A Motor paralysis
    - B Hyperactive tendon reflexes
    - C Loss of pain sensation
    - D Loss of temperature sensation
    - E Loss of position sense

37. **Resting tremor is a characteristic symptom of:**
    - A Cerebellar disorders
    - B Temporal lobe epilepsy
    - C Parkinsonism
    - D Alcoholism
    - E Thyrotoxicosis

38. **Prostaglandins:**
    - A Occur only in the prostate
    - B Mediate pseudo-hermaphroditism
    - C Cause pseudo-neurotic schizophrenia
    - D Are increased in prostitutes
    - E Have been postulated as synaptic transmitters in the brain

39. Recognized precipitants of convulsive seizures include:
A Anoxia
B Electrical stimulation
C Barbiturate withdrawal
D Flickering lights
E Diazepam administration

40. Echolalia is a recognized symptom of:
A Severe mental subnormality
B Parkinsonism
C Catatonia
D Obsessional neurosis
E Dementia

41. The name of Erik H. Erikson is typically associated with:
A Eight ages of man
B Study of childhood in two American Indian tribes
C A theory of infantile sexuality
D Neurosurgical advances
E Aversion treatment of alcoholism

42. The grasp reflex is a recognized symptom of:
A Depressive psychosis
B Cerebellar disorders
C Hypomania
D Widespread disorder of cerebral cortex
E Frontal lobe lesions

43. The following drugs cause pupillary dilatation:
A Morphia
B LSD
C Atropine
D Parasympatholytics
E Sympathomimetics

44. Major factors in maintaining the level of deleterious dominant genes in the population include:
    A Natural selection
    B Sex-linkage
    C The occurrence of fresh mutations
    D Delay of onset of harmful effects until after commencement of the reproductive period
    E Variability in the manifestations of the gene

45. Characteristic clinical signs of cerebellar dysfunction include:
    A Ataxia
    B Hypertonia
    C Dysdiadochokinesia
    D Nystagmus
    E Nominal aphasia

46. Recognized features of alcohol withdrawal include:
    A Epileptic seizures
    B Constricted pupils
    C Bradycardia
    D Vivid dreams
    E Absence of sweating

47. Characteristic symptoms of catatonic schizophrenia include:
    A Catalepsy
    B Stereotyped postures
    C Negativism
    D Stupor
    E Cog-wheel rigidity

48. *Descending* fibres of the spinal cord are the main components of the following tracts:
    A Dorsal columns
    B Spinocerebellar tract
    C Vestibulospinal tract
    D Rubrospinal tract
    E Pyramidal tract

49. **Examples of conditions characteristically transmitted by polygenic (multifactorial) inheritance include:**
    A ABO blood groups
    B Intelligence
    C Harelip–cleft-palate syndrome
    D Huntington's chorea
    E Tuberous sclerosis

50. **Characteristic symptoms of obsessional neurosis include:**
    A Thought blocking
    B Retardation of thinking
    C Primary delusions
    D Perseveration
    E Thought alienation

51. **The following statements concerning lower motor neurone lesions are correct:**
    A They result from damage to the anterior horn cell
    B They result from damage to the ventral root of the mixed spinal nerve
    C They result in increased tone of the affected muscles
    D They result from thiamine deficiency
    E They result from cerebro-vascular accidents

52. **Side-effects of tricyclic antidepressants include:**
    A Blurred vision
    B Dry mouth
    C Constipation
    D Tremor
    E Urinary retention

53. **Mutism is significantly associated with:**
    A Depressive stupor
    B Catatonic stupor
    C Hysteria
    D Frontal lobe syndrome
    E Korsakoff's psychosis

54. **Systematic desensitization includes:**
    A Anxiety reduction by relaxation techniques
    B Use of a hierarchy
    C Desensitization in imagination
    D Flooding
    E Desensitization *in vivo*

55. **Characteristic symptoms of dementia include:**
    A Deterioration of the personality
    B Loss of memory
    C Loss of intelligence
    D Auditory hallucinations
    E Delusions of persecution

56. **Lithium carbonate therapy is appropriate treatment for:**
    A Hyponatraemia
    B Hypothyroidism
    C Dementia
    D Prophylaxis of bipolar manic-depressive psychosis
    E Hypomania

57. **Auditory hallucinations are recognized symptoms of:**
    A Depressive psychosis
    B Alcoholic hallucinosis
    C Sensory deprivation
    D Temporal lobe stimulation
    E Cerebral atrophy

58. **Lesions in the spinal cord causing loss of pain sensation include:**
    A Tabes dorsalis
    B Brown–Sequard syndrome
    C Syringomyelia
    D Acute poliomyelitis
    E Peripheral neuritis

59. **Recognized functions of the glossopharyngeal nerve include:**
- A Taste sensation from the anterior third of the tongue
- B Innervation of the parotid gland
- C Sensation from the pharynx
- D Innervation of the muscles of mastication
- E Innervation of the superficial muscles of the face

60. **Characteristic features of Cushing's syndrome include:**
- A Truncal obesity
- B Hypotension
- C Menorrhagia
- D Proximal muscle weakness
- E Osteoporosis

Paper 5

1. Characteristic features of Parkinson's disease include:
   - A Cog-wheel rigidity
   - B Resting tremor
   - C Bradykinesia
   - D Mask-like facies
   - E Choreiform movements

2. Destruction of the right optic tract results in:
   - A Left homonymous hemianopia
   - B Paralysis of right lateral gaze
   - C Bitemporal hemianopia
   - D Blindness for objects in the left half of each field of vision
   - E Loss of visual function in the right halves of both retinae

3. Characteristic features of thyrotoxicosis include:
   - A Bradycardia
   - B Excessive sweating
   - C A preference for cold weather
   - D Weight gain
   - E Anorexia

4. Visual hallucinations are recognized symptoms of:
   - A Delirium tremens
   - B Atropine poisoning
   - C Schizophrenia
   - D Temporal lobe tumour
   - E Hydrocephalus

5. **Learned helplessness:**
   A Is a concept introduced by Seligman
   B Has been measured in experimental work on dogs
   C Has been invoked as a contributing factor to depressive illness
   D Results in subsequent failure to escape from stressful situations
   E Is the main cause of passive homosexuality

6. **The following statements concerning innate releasing mechanisms are correct:**
   A They respond to the overall total of the stimuli accompanying a certain relevant situation
   B They respond to specific sign stimuli
   C Gestalt perception by the organism is necessary in order to produce a response
   D Releasers consist of morphological structures
   E Releasers consist of innate motor patterns

7. **The Camberwell Register:**
   A Is a cumulative psychiatric case register
   B Is a measure of the validity of diagnosis
   C Gives an estimate of period prevalence
   D Is a list of Maudsley graduates
   E Gives an estimate of incidence

8. **Delirium tremens is characterized by:**
   A Confusion
   B Disorders of perception
   C Hypersomnia
   D Delusions
   E Impairment of recent memory

9. **The following statements concerning the Median are correct:**
   - A It is the point of maximum frequency density
   - B Half of the items in a distribution have a value equal to or above it
   - C It is unaffected by the value of extreme items in the distribution
   - D In calculating it, every value in the distribution is used
   - E It is the most frequently occurring value in a distribution

10. **Characteristics in which man differs from other mammals include:**
    - A Increase in behavioural versatility
    - B Decrease in instinctive motor patterns
    - C Increase in specialization of innate releasing mechanisms
    - D Decrease in exploratory learning
    - E Ability to maintain an existence in a wider range of environments

11. **The following statements concerning percentiles are correct:**
    - A They are fractiles
    - B They relate to hundredths of the way through a distribution
    - C They are typically useful as 'cut-off' values
    - D They are typically useful for measuring statistical significance
    - E They are typically useful for measuring dispersion

12. **Recognized features of the triple-X (XXX) constitution include:**
    - A Characteristically higher than average intelligence
    - B Chromatin-positive smears
    - C Inheritance as an X-linked dominant
    - D An obviously abnormal phenotype
    - E A pathognomic EEG abnormality

13. The following are concepts from psychoanalytic theory:
  A Sublimation
  B Imprinting
  C The unconscious mind
  D Risky shift
  E Group conformity

14. Characteristics of hebephrenic schizophrenia include:
  A Disturbance of short-term memory
  B Impaired rapport
  C Disturbance of affect
  D Disturbance of thought form
  E Disturbance of behaviour

15. Recognized consequences of hypothyroidism include:
  A Bradycardia
  B Delay in relaxation of tendon reflexes
  C Lethargy
  D Rapid speech
  E Increased metabolic rate

16. The following statements are true of the cell membrane during the resting state:
  A Intracellular sodium is greater than extracellular sodium
  B Intracellular K^+ is greater than extracellular K^+
  C Intracellular Cl^- is greater than extracellular Cl^-
  D Membrane potential is greater than –200 mV
  E The membrane is polarized

17. Characteristic symptoms of acute brain syndrome include:
  A Disorientation
  B Short-term memory disturbance
  C Confusion
  D Excessive appetite
  E Global amnesia

18. **Desensitization typically involves the use of:**
   A Apomorphine
   B Flooding
   C Electric shocks
   D Relaxation
   E Token economies

19. **The following structures have a significant involvement in the control of respiration:**
   A Carotid body
   B Phrenic nerves
   C Vagus nerve
   D Hypothalamus
   E Reticular formation

20. **Vegetative depressive symptoms typically include:**
   A Constipation
   B Knight's move thinking
   C Thought broadcasting
   D Weight loss
   E Loss of libido

21. **Broadbent's filter model:**
   A Is concerned with selective attention
   B Explains the mechanism of the blood–brain barrier
   C Is a concept from cybernetics
   D Accounts for the development of phobias
   E Has been implicated in the pathogenesis of schizophrenia

22. **The oculomotor nerve innervates the following muscles:**
   A Inferior oblique
   B Lateral rectus
   C Superior oblique
   D Superior rectus
   E Ciliary muscle

23. **Disorders characterized by autosomal chromosome anomalies include:**
   A Down's syndrome (mongolism)
   B Cri-du-chat syndrome
   C Red-green colour blindness
   D Partial deletion of number five chromosome
   E Klinefelter's syndrome

24. **Recognized features of upper motor neurone lesions of the facial nerve include:**
   A Trigeminal neuralgia
   B Sparing of the upper part of the face from paralysis
   C Paralysis of the muscles of the lower part of the face
   D An apparent absence of paralysis during involuntary contraction of the muscles of facial expression
   E Bell's palsy

25. **Behaviour modification procedures include:**
   A Modelling
   B Aversion therapy
   C Flooding
   D Response prevention
   E Operant conditioning

26. **Characteristics of weighted aggregative cost indexes include:**
   A The use of Base 100
   B Negative skew
   C Multiplication of the prices by the selected weights
   D Adding the products
   E Bimodal distribution

27. **The following substances interact with monoamine oxidase inhibitors:**
   A Tricyclic antidepressants
   B Methyldopa
   C Barbiturates
   D Tyramine
   E Cheese

28. **Compliance to authority:**
- A Has been investigated by Milgram
- B In the experimental situation exceeds that predicted by both laymen and psychiatrists
- C Is typically stronger in women than in men in the experimental situation
- D Caused the ulcers in Brady's executive monkeys
- E Depends on the proximity of the subject to the victim

29. **The following statements are true of the psychogalvanic reflex (PGR); (Galvanic Skin Response):**
- A Speed of habituation of the PGR is negatively correlated with ratings of anxiety
- B There is a positive correlation between the frequency of spontaneous fluctuations and ratings of anxiety
- C Spontaneous fluctuations are decreased in number in patients with conversion hysteria
- D Spontaneous fluctuations are decreased in number in patients during the phenomenon of derealization
- E A characteristic pattern is diagnostic of schizophrenia

30. **The parts visible on the outer surface of an undamaged post-mortem brain include:**
- A Amygdaloid nuclei
- B Interventricular foramen
- C Optic chiasma
- D Dura mater
- E Trigeminal nerve roots

31. **Instrumental conditioning includes:**
- A Reward training
- B Escape training
- C Avoidance training
- D Operant conditioning
- E Classical conditioning

32. **Recognized features of the stimulation of the parasympathetic nervous system include:**
   A Penile erection
   B Ejaculation
   C Pupillary constriction
   D Salivation
   E Bronchiolar dilatation

33. **Factors influencing a time series include:**
   A Seasonal variation
   B The trend
   C Random variation
   D Correlation coefficient
   E The arithmetic mean

34. **Succinylcholine chloride (Scoline):**
   A Is a hypnotic
   B Should be given in the same syringe as methohexitone or thiopentone
   C Is hydrolysed by acetylcholinesterase
   D Is responsible for degradation of acetylcholine
   E Is hydrolysed by pseudocholinesterase

35. **Structures contributing to the maintenance of decerebrate rigidity in the cat include:**
   A Reticular formation of the lower brain stem
   B Vestibular nuclei
   C The eighth cranial nerve
   D Oculomotor nuclei
   E Olfactory nerve

36. **Cognitive dissonance:**
   A Is a theory of Festinger
   B Is a recognized cause of the effectiveness of electroconvulsive therapy
   C Is a theory of attitude change
   D Relies on imprinting
   E Follows a choice between two similar alternatives

37. **Lesions of the middle part of the optic chiasma:**

A Result in blocking of the visual impulses from the temporal halves of each retina
B Are a recognized complication of pituitary tumour
C Are a recognized complication of craniopharyngioma
D Result in defects of the temporal field of each eye
E Result in binasal hemianopia

38. **Recognized features of atropine poisoning include:**

A Blocking of vagal action
B Slowing of heart rate
C Psychosis
D Dry mouth
E Pupillary constriction

39. **Recognized therapeutic levels of lithium:**

A Are between 0.6 and 1.2 mEq/l
B Are 3–6 mEq/l
C May result in a non-toxic goitre in a significant number of cases
D May result in fine tremor in a significant percentage of cases
E Are monitored by urine tests in preference to blood tests

40. **The following are amino acids:**

A L-phenylalanine
B L-tyrosine
C Serotonin
D Noradrenaline
E Dopamine

41. **The following statements concerning criminology are correct:**
   A Peak incidence of criminal convictions in males is 18–24 years
   B In the United Kingdom, the female incidence of criminal conviction is equal to the male incidence
   C There is a significant association between sociopathy and alcoholism
   D MMPI results on psychopaths are typically within the normal range
   E In the United Kingdom, the incidence of delinquent behaviour among young Chinese immigrant girls exceeds that among young West Indian immigrant girls

42. **Enkephalins:**
   A Are cerebral beta lipoproteins
   B Have been postulated as neurotransmitters
   C Are monoamines
   D Are morphia-like in action
   E Are blocked by nalorphine

43. **Structures characteristically involved in conversion hysteria include:**
   A Endocrine systems
   B Somatic motor nervous system
   C Somatic sensory nervous system
   D Sympathetic nervous system
   E Parasympathetic nervous system

44. **Depression is a recognized complication of treatment with the following drugs:**
   A Progestogen–oestrogen formulations
   B Alpha-methyl-dopa
   C Pyridoxine
   D Thiamine
   E Diazepam

45. Characteristic features of manic-depressive psychosis include:
   A Disturbance of affect
   B Delusional perception
   C Primary delusions
   D Thought-blocking
   E Initial onset below age 25 years in the majority of cases

46. Factors conditioning the entry of substances from the bloodstream to the brain include:
   A Carrier-mediated transport mechanisms
   B Membrane permeability
   C Concentration gradient
   D Lipid solubility
   E Stereospecificity

47. Recognized features of high introversion include:
   A High state of cortical arousal
   B Raised sedation threshold to sodium amytal
   C Higher speed of acquiring conditioned reflexes
   D Poor long-term memory
   E Better short-term memory

48. Typical features of Wernicke's encephalopathy include:
   A Ganser symptoms
   B Confusion
   C Nystagmus
   D Ophthalmoplegia
   E Effective treatment by thiamine

49. Characteristic symptoms of hypomania include:
   A Circumstantiality
   B Flight of ideas
   C Perseveration
   D Pressure of speech
   E Elevation of mood

50. **The following statements concerning Alzheimer's disease are correct:**
   A Plaques are mainly in the cortex
   B There is an increased incidence in Down's syndrome (Mongolism)
   C It is characteristically associated with cardiac enlargement
   D Neurofibrillary tangles occur predominantly in the cerebellum rather than in the cerebrum
   E It is a recognized cause of the Sturge–Weber syndrome

51. **The following are catecholamines:**
   A Dihydroxyphenylalanine
   B Dopamine
   C Adrenaline
   D Serotonin
   E Imipramine

52. **Temporal lobe epilepsy is significantly associated with:**
   A Bipolar affective illness
   B Ammon's horn sclerosis
   C 3 per second spikes and waves on electroencephalogram
   D Schizophreniform psychosis
   E Déjà vu experiences

53. **Enzymes involved in the formation of catecholamines include:**
   A Dopamine beta hydroxylase
   B Dopa decarboxylase
   C Monoamine oxidase
   D Tyrosine hydroxylase
   E Phenylalanine hydroxylase

54. **Recognized studies of the relative contributions of heredity and environment to intelligence include:**
   - A Studies of foster-children
   - B Work with twins
   - C Correlations between relatives
   - D Cell culture tests
   - E Prenatal genetical diagnosis

55. **On examination of the visual fields:**
   - A Bitemporal hemianopia is indicative of chiasmatic compression
   - B The finding of a right homonymous hemianopia would be consistent with a space-occupying lesion in the left occipital lobe
   - C Bilateral concentric constriction of the fields can only be due to conversion hysteria
   - D A central scotoma is consistent with a lesion of the lateral geniculate body
   - E An upper quadrantic homonymous defect would suggest a temporal lobe lesion

56. **Suxamethonium (Scoline):**
   - A Is extremely irritant to the tissues in the event of extravenous injection
   - B Is a competitive blocker of neuro-muscular transmission
   - C Has a prolonged action in liver failure
   - D Is known to cause muscle pain post-operatively
   - E Is known to cause bradycardia when administered intermittently

57. **According to Freudian psychology:**
   - A All of the energy used for performing the work of the personality is obtained from the instincts
   - B An instinct is the mental representative of a bodily need
   - C The extrovert is slow at imprinting
   - D The energy from a blocked cathexis distributes itself among new activities
   - E The superego is formed out of the ego

58. **Projective techniques of personality assessment:**
   A Have been validated by Eysenck
   B Encourage freedom and diversity of response
   C Form the traditional tool of the psychometrist
   D Are independent of the personality of the examiner
   E Provide objective measures of performance

59. **Disturbances of the body image are significantly associated with:**
   A Anorexia nervosa
   B Amputation
   C Gerstmann's syndrome
   D Sociopathic personality disorder
   E Lithium therapy

60. **Features of increased intracranial pressure include:**
   A Headache
   B Vomiting
   C Papilloedema
   D Slowing of the pulse rate
   E Slowing of the respiratory rate

Membership Examination Questions

Paper 6

1. Recognized symptoms of anxiety neurosis include:
   - A Breathlessness
   - B Sweating of palms
   - C Dizziness
   - D Chest pain relieved by glyceryl trinitrate
   - E Burning on micturition

2. Dynamic causes of anxiety neurosis are recognized to include:
   - A Sublimation
   - B Excessive repression
   - C Homosexual libidinal drives
   - D Aggressive drives and their derivative emotions and fantasies
   - E The threatened emergence into consciousness of forbidden repressed mental contents

3. Recognized symptoms of hysterical neurosis, dissociative type, include:
   - A Somnambulism
   - B Amnesia
   - C Schizophrenic thought disorder
   - D Fugue states
   - E Multiple personalities

4. Recognized signs of hysterical neurosis, conversion type, include:
   A Belle indifférence
   B Pathognomic brain wave changes
   C Constricted pupils
   D Dilated pupils
   E Akathisia

5. Recognized treatments for phobic neurosis include:
   A Flooding
   B Reciprocal inhibition
   C Amine depletion
   D Systematic desensitization
   E ECT

6. The following persons are recognized as having made significant contributions to the understanding of schizophrenia:
   A Emil Kraepelin
   B John Bowlby
   C Eugen Bleuler
   D Washington Irving
   E Harry Stack Sullivan

7. Object relations theoreticians include:
   A Schreber
   B Ronald Fairbairn
   C H. Guntrip
   D J. Piaget
   E E. Robbins

8. Recognized symptoms and signs of simple schizophrenia include:
   A Delusions of persecution
   B Negativism
   C Marked thought disorder
   D Deterioration of the personality
   E Loss of ambition

9. **Recognized symptoms and signs of catatonic schizophrenia include:**
   A Frontal headache
   B Abnormal motor behaviour
   C Stupor
   D Excitement
   E Delusions of grandeur

10. **Recognized causes of paranoid delusions include:**
   A Schizophrenia
   B Affective illness
   C Amphetamine addiction
   D Alcoholism
   E Social isolation with deafness

11. **The following drugs are tricyclic antidepressants:**
   A Doxepin
   B Phenelzine
   C Tranylcypromine
   D Methylphenidate
   E Isocarboxazid

12. **The following statements concerning monoamine oxidase inhibitors are correct:**
   A MAO inhibitors can be safely given in combination with tricyclics provided that there is no evidence of latent hypertension
   B MAO inhibitors are generally more effective than tricyclic derivatives in endogenous depression
   C MAO inhibitors are used mainly for patients who have not responded to tricyclic antidepressants
   D Hypertensive encephalopathy has resulted from toxic interactions involving all commonly-used MAO inhibitors *except* tranylcypromine
   E The combination of tranylcypromine and dextroamphetamine is effective in the treatment of schizoaffective psychosis

13. **Recognized features of antisocial personality disorder include:**
   - A Commoner over the age of forty years
   - B Self-injury
   - C Good response to analytically oriented psychotherapy
   - D Good response to chemotherapy
   - E School and work accomplishments exceed those which innate abilities promise

14. **The following statements are true of Wernicke's encephalopathy:**
   - A It is caused by a deficiency of thiamine
   - B It invariably progresses to Korsakoff's psychosis despite prompt treatment
   - C Eye movement paralyses indicate that it is too late for treatment
   - D The most important aspect of treatment is adequate sedation
   - E It is significantly associated with alcoholism

15. **Characteristic features of Jakob–Creutzfeldt disease include:**
   - A Transmission by an agent, presumably a slow virus
   - B Myoclonic jerks
   - C Normal electroencephalogram
   - D Spontaneous cure
   - E Rapidly progressive dementia

16. **Characteristic features of anorexia nervosa include:**
   - A Lack of *interest* in food
   - B Disturbance of body image
   - C Amenorrhoea
   - D Compulsive masturbation in the male
   - E Reduction of physical activity

17. **The following statements are true of chlorpromazine:**
    A It is more sedative than is trifluoperazine
    B It is more likely to produce *hypotension* than is perphenazine
    C It is less likely to produce Parkinsonism than is haloperidol
    D As an injection it is less painful than haloperidol
    E It is less likely to cause photosensitivity than is haloperidol

18. **The following statements are true of acute dystonic reactions to phenothiazines:**
    A The majority are hysterical in nature
    B Treatment by parenteral injection of an antiparkinson agent is effective in the majority of cases
    C They occur only in the presence of schizophrenia
    D Treatment by administering higher doses of phenothiazines is effective in the majority of cases
    E They do not occur unless antipsychotic medication has been given for a long period

19. **Behaviour therapy is a recognized treatment for the following disorders:**
    A Phobias
    B Obsessive-compulsive neuroses
    C Impotence
    D Bipolar affective disorder
    E Acute schizophrenia

20. **The following statements concerning electroconvulsive therapy are correct:**
    A It results in cure in the majority of cases of chronic schizophrenia
    B Additional current, greater than that necessary to produce a convulsion, results in greater therapeutic effect
    C Therapeutic effect is directly proportional to memory loss
    D It is an effective treatment for pseudoneurotic schizophrenia
    E It is necessary for a *cortical* seizure to occur in order to obtain a therapeutic response

21. Signs of physiological withdrawal from alcohol include:
- A Absence of alcohol on the breath
- B Sweating
- C Hyperreflexia
- D Increasing tachycardia
- E Hyperventilation

22. The following statements concerning attempted suicide are correct:
- A The events immediately preceding the attempt do not have any bearing on the underlying problem
- B Every patient who attempts must be admitted to a psychiatric hospital
- C The probabilities of future fatal attempts are greater in young healthy females than in elderly sick males
- D The seriousness of the intent can be clearly evaluated from the choice of the method used
- E The probabilities of future fatal attempts are greater in alcoholics

23. Medical complications of chronic alcoholism include:
- A Polyneuritis
- B Cerebellar degeneration
- C Pancreatitis
- D Cardiomyopathy
- E Neurofibromatosis

24. The following statements concerning theories of the aetiology of schizophrenia are correct:
- A Gregory Bateson described 'double-bind'
- B T. Lidz described 'skew and schism'
- C Wynne and Singer described 'family transactions'
- D John Wing described the 'special strategy that a person invents in order to live in an unliveable situation
- E R.D. Laing described 'dimethyltryptamine'

25. **A paper published by J. Snow in 1855 concerned the 'Broad Street Pump Incident'. The following statements are correct:**
A It related to an outbreak of smallpox
B The epidemic spared the region of the Broad Street pump
C This incident followed Pasteur's work leading to the germ theory of disease
D Dismantling of the Broad Street pump brought the epidemic under control
E Epidemiological inquiry produced data about the association among variables

26. **The following groups have a higher incidence of mental illness than does the general population:**
A Separated or divorced
B Professional and managerial class
C Widowed
D Biological children of schizophrenic parents
E Refugees

27. **The authors in column I published the studies in column II:**

	I	II
A	Erich Lindemann	'Cocoanut Grove Fire'
B	Grad and Sainsbury	'A Mind that Found Itself'
C	C.W. Beers	'Suicide and Hospitalization Rates in Chichester'
D	G.W. Brown *et al.*	'Schizophrenia and Social Care'
E	G. Caplan	'Principles of Preventive Psychiatry'

28. **The following statements concerning community psychiatry are correct:**
    A Elimination of schizophrenia by mental health education is a realistic goal
    B Avoidance of institutionalization prevents any loss of volition in schizophrenia
    C Community-based services are invariably less expensive than institution-based services
    D The most seriously ill have tended to be neglected
    E The value of a self-help programme is directly proportional to the academic qualifications of its members

29. **In order to be considered competent to make a will (to have testamentary capacity) a person must know:**
    A The date and correct address
    B The nature and extent of the property of which he is about to dispose
    C That he is not certifiable under the Mental Health Act
    D The names and identity of persons who are to be the objects of his bounty
    E His relation towards persons who are to be the objects of his bounty

30. **Characteristic features of the hyperkinetic syndrome of childhood include:**
    A Distractability
    B Short attention span
    C Impulsivity
    D Enuresis
    E Tics

31. **Recognized features of tics (sudden, frequent, purposeless movements) include:**
    A Usual onset before age four years
    B A preponderance in girls
    C Occurrence predominantly in those of below average intelligence
    D A good response to haloperidol
    E Characteristic association with visual hallucinations

32. **Recognized stages in the life histories of pre-schizophrenic individuals include:**
    - A Early timidity and shyness
    - B Improving social performance
    - C Loss of peer relationships in adolescence
    - D Rise in social status
    - E Migration into urban areas

33. **The following statements concerning schizophrenia are correct:**
    - A Heston (1966) found a lower incidence of schizophrenia in the adopted-away children of chronic schizophrenic mothers, than in a control group of non-psychotic parentage
    - B Rosenthal *et al.* (1968) found that the children of schizophrenic parents suffered an excess of schizophrenic disorder, even when adopted away
    - C Adoption studies prove that environmental factors do not contribute to the aetiology of schizophrenia
    - D Slater and Cowie (1971) put forward the monogenic theory of the inheritance
    - E Gottesman and Shields (1972, 1973) put forward the polygenic theory of the inheritance

34. **The following statements concerning schizophrenia are correct:**
    - A Amphetamines have been found to cause relief of symptoms in the majority of patients
    - B L-DOPA has been found to cause behavioural worsening in schizophrenic patients
    - C Phenothiazines act as antagonists at CNS dopamine receptors
    - D Neuroleptics cause an increase in circulating levels of the pituitary hormone, prolactin
    - E Neuroleptic drugs have high lipid solubility

35. **The following statements concerning treatment of schizophrenia are correct:**
   - A Benzhexol prevents the weight gain resulting from chlorpromazine use
   - B It is recognized as good treatment practice to change the type of drug daily during the acute stages
   - C Electroconvulsive therapy remains the treatment of choice for an acute episode
   - D Leff and Wing (1971) found that the relapse rate of patients on an active drug was less than the relapse rate of those on placebo
   - E Patients excluded from Leff and Wing's trial (1971) on account of poor prognosis did badly, even though kept on their original medications

36. **The following statements concerning the history of psychiatry are correct:**
   - A Philippe Pinel wrote 'The Myth of Mental Illness'
   - B Emil Kraepelin separated dementia praecox from manic-depressive psychosis
   - C Pierre Janet discovered that traumatic memories which the patient had forgotten could be recovered during hypnosis
   - D Adolf Meyer wrote 'Characteristics of Total Institutions'
   - E Melanie Klein wrote 'Childhood and Society'

37. **The following statements concerning suicide rates in England and Wales are correct:**
   - A The rates were higher during the two world wars than during the period between the wars
   - B Over the years 1900–1960, rates for women increased to a greater extent than did rates for men
   - C Over the years 1955–1970, the rate for males fell
   - D Over the years 1955–1970, the rate for females rose
   - E The change described in the correct answer to 'C' above was due principally to an alteration in the carbon monoxide content of domestic gas

38. **Suicide rates (England and Wales) are higher in the following groups than in the general population:**
   A Alcoholics
   B Drug addicts
   C Patients with personality disorders
   D Patients with reactive depression
   E Female Maltese visitors

39. **The following statements concerning parasuicide (attempted suicide) in the United Kingdom are correct:**
   A The commonest mode is attempted hanging
   B The act occurs under the influence of alcohol in more than 25% of cases
   C Persons with personality disorders have a higher rate than does the general population
   D There is a significant positive correlation between the toxicity sustained by the patient and the severity of any underlying psychological illness
   E Social workers have no place in crisis intervention

40. **Recognized predictors of the likelihood of a further parasuicide (attempted suicide) act in an individual include:**
   A Membership of Social Class V
   B Dependence on drugs
   C Unemployment at the time of the act
   D History of criminal behaviour
   E Use of a particularly hazardous method for the first parasuicide

41. The following statements concerning suicide and parasuicide (attempted suicide) in the United Kingdom are correct:

A The period of greatest danger following a parasuicide is in the few months following the act itself

B Crisis intervention (for example, by Telephone Samaritans) significantly reduces the prevailing parasuicide rate

C The clientele of Telephone Samaritans approximates more to the population of parasuicides than of suicides

D For women, parasuicide rates are more than ten times the suicide rates

E The relative excess of parasuicide to suicide is greater for young women than for older men

42. The following statements concerning mental handicap in the United Kingdom are correct:

A The prevalence of moderate and severe mental retardation is greater than 50/1000 population

B Subnormality is commoner in females than in males

C Down's syndrome (Mongolism) occurs in approximately 1.6/1000 live births

D The incidence of Down's syndrome for 45-year-old mothers is approximately 1 in 2300 births

E Down's syndrome occurs in approximately 8.5% of the subnormal (IQ below 70) population

43. The following statements concerning cerebral palsy are correct:

A The disorder progressively worsens

B Low intelligence is a characteristic feature

C It is significantly associated with premature delivery

D It is significantly associated with chromosomal abnormalities

E Patients who suffer from spastic tetraplegia are usually the least mentally handicapped

44. **The following statements concerning phenylketonuria are correct:**
   A There is an excess of the enzyme phenylalanine hydroxylase
   B The Guthrie test is a screening test for this illness
   C Blood phenylalanine is elevated in affected babies
   D Adequate treatment includes a diet high in phenylalanine hydroxylase
   E Convulsions occur in about one-third of all cases

45. **The following statements concerning infantile autism are correct**
   A Usual onset is after the age of 30 months
   B It is commoner in boys than in girls
   C Aetiology is clear in the majority of cases
   D If one child is autistic then the siblings are also autistic, in the majority of cases
   E There is a well established genetic link between childhood autism and adult schizophrenia

46. **Aggressive behaviour (conduct disorder) is commoner in:**
   A Boys
   B Socially deprived children
   C Children from families disrupted by marital discord
   D Children who are educationally retarded
   E Children from Social Classes I and II

47. **Recognized uses of amphetamines, in good clinical practice, include the treatment of:**
   A Neurotic depression
   B Narcolepsy
   C Schizophrenia
   D Hyperkinetic syndrome of childhood
   E Obesity

48. **Factors significantly associated with an increased risk of alcoholism include:**
   A Divorce
   B Jewish religion
   C Employment in the sale of alcoholic drinks
   D Social Class III
   E Parental alcoholism

49. **Workers who have made significant contributions in statistical analysis of affective disorders include:**
   A Hamilton and White (1959)
   B Kiloh and Garside (1963)
   C Kendell (1968)
   D Meyer and Chesser (1970)
   E Eysenck (1970)

50. **The following statements concerning studies of manic-depressive psychosis are correct:**
   A Kraepelin (1921) described two distinct disease entities: bipolar and unipolar
   B Slater (1936) proposed transmission by a single autosomal dominant gene with reduced penetrance
   C Leonhard (1959, 1962) proposed that the illness was a single disease entity
   D Perris (1966) reported different heredity patterns between bipolar and unipolar probands
   E Winokur (1969) proposed that an X-linked dominant gene was a major aetiological factor

51. **Recognized causes of cerebral hypoxia include:**
   A Carbon monoxide poisoning
   B Bronchopneumonia
   C Myocardial infarction
   D High altitudes
   E Chronic bronchitis

52. **Recognized features of acute intermittent porphyria include:**
   A Transmission as a Mendelian recessive
   B Precipitation of acute attacks by barbiturates
   C Colour change of freshly voided urine on exposure to light
   D Acute abdominal pain
   E Mental confusion

53. **Disorders in which there is a preponderance of women include:**
   A Neurotic depression
   B Senile dementia
   C Transsexualism
   D Latah
   E Criminal behaviour

54. **The following statements concerning the psychobiology of disease are correct:**
   A Dunbar believed that particular character or personality traits were associated with particular diseases
   B Alexander stressed the importance of life events and social readjustments
   C Lipowski stressed the importance of consultation psychiatry in psychosomatic medicine
   D Holmes and Rahe described central control in endocrine systems
   E Kubler-Ross pioneered the use of biofeedback

55. **The following statements concerning Folie à Deux are correct:**
   A A dominant delusional person induces a parallel delusional development in a dependent one
   B If the two are separated, the dominant one recovers quickly
   C If the two are separated, the dependent one recovers quickly
   D A majority exhibit persecutory paranoid delusions
   E The persons involved live in intimate contact, in the majority of cases

56. **Symptoms commoner in the bereaved than in married groups include:**
   A Excessive sleep
   B Loss of appetite
   C Trembling
   D Persistent fears
   E Nightmares

57. **The following workers have made significant contributions to the understanding of anorexia nervosa:**
   - A A.H. Crisp
   - B P.M. Yap
   - C G.F.M. Russell
   - D E.M. Jellinek
   - E Hilde Bruch

58. **The following show an increased incidence of anorexia nervosa:**
   - A Social Classes I and II
   - B Males
   - C Geriatric patients
   - D Daughters of placid fathers
   - E Delinquent girls

59. **The following statements concerning lithium are correct:**
   - A Rate of removal from the body is increased by the use of thiazide diuretics
   - B The management of lithium intoxication should include restriction of sodium intake
   - C Blood levels do not become maximal until later than six hours after ingestion
   - D The average half-life in the body in young adults is approximately forty hours
   - E Lithium ion does not bind to plasma proteins

60. **The syndromes in the left-hand column are correctly paired with the labels in the right-hand column**

A	The giving of approximate answers	Ganser's syndrome
B	Identification of a known person as a double or imposter	Capgras' syndrome
C	Recognition of a double of oneself	Autoscopic syndrome
D	Irrational belief of being loved	Clérambault's syndrome
E	Repeatedly feigning serious illness	Munchausen's syndrome

Paper 7

1. **Recognized symptoms of anxiety neurosis include:**
   A Terminal insomnia
   B Delusions
   C Heartburn
   D Headache
   E Backache

2. **Recognized treatments for anxiety neurosis include:**
   A Progressive relaxation exercises
   B Transcendental meditation
   C Hypnotic suggestion
   D Electroconvulsive therapy
   E The minor tranquillizers

3. **Recognized treatments for hysterical neurosis, dissociative type, include:**
   A Exploratory and supportive psychotherapy
   B ECT
   C Hypnosis
   D Sensory deprivation
   E Sodium amytal interview

4. **Recognized treatments for hysterical neurosis, conversion type, include:**
   A Flooding
   B Psychoanalysis
   C Hypnotic suggestion
   D Supportive therapy
   E Coffee enemas

5. **Recognized treatments for obsessive-compulsive neurosis include:**
   A Analytically oriented therapy
   B Response prevention
   C Modeling
   D Clomipramine
   E ECT

6. **Psychiatrists recognized for their descriptions of the symptoms and signs of schizophrenia include:**
   A H.J. Eysenck
   B Eugen Bleuler
   C Donald Winnicott
   D Kurt Schneider
   E H. Guntrip

7. **Workers recognized for socioepidemiological studies of schizophrenia include:**
   A R.E.L. Faris and H.W. Dunham
   B L. Srole *et al.*
   C A.B. Hollingshead
   D Melanie Klein
   E H. Guntrip

8. **In 1898 Kraepelin organized the signs and symptoms of dementia praecox into clinical syndromes, now known as:**
   A Borderline syndrome
   B Catatonic schizophrenia
   C Hebephrenic schizophrenia
   D Paranoid schizophrenia
   E Simple schizophrenia

9. **Recognized symptoms and signs of paranoid schizophrenia include:**
   A Delusions of persecution
   B Early morning waking
   C Pressure of speech
   D Disturbance of recent memory
   E Marked thought disorder

10. The following workers are recognized for their research into the distinction between unipolar and bipolar affective disorders
    - A K. Leonhard
    - B O. Rank
    - C O. Fenichel
    - D J. Angst
    - E G. Winokur

11. The following statements concerning the administration of tricyclic antidepressants are correct:
    - A Initial therapeutic response is usually evident within twenty-four hours of commencing treatment
    - B Doses are standardized and there is therefore no need to individualize dosage to suit the patient
    - C A suitable starting dose of amitriptyline or imipramine for a geriatric patient is 200 mg daily
    - D Induction of cardiac arrhythmia is less common in the elderly
    - E Adverse effects from sudden withdrawal of tricyclics include nausea and vomiting

12. Lithium carbonate is recognized as useful in:
    - A Treatment of acute mania
    - B Prophylaxis of recurrent mania
    - C Prophylaxis of bipolar affective illness
    - D Treatment of severe acute depressive illness
    - E Treatment of acute paranoid schizophrenia

13. Recognized causes of profound change of character (personality) include:
    - A Vascular disease of the brain
    - B Alzheimer's disease
    - C Heavy metal intoxication
    - D Neoplastic disease
    - E General paresis: tertiary neurosyphilis

14. **Factors recognized to be involved in the aetiology of post-operative delirium include:**
    A Metabolic imbalances
    B Anaesthetic effects
    C Infection, with fever
    D Sensory deprivation
    E Withdrawal from alcohol

15. **Characteristic features of chronic subdural haematoma include:**
    A A clearly remembered traumatic episode
    B Pathognomic mental state
    C Invariably normal findings on computerized tomography
    D Surgical evacuation of no benefit
    E Schizophreniform psychosis

16. **Workers recognized for research into duodenal ulcer disease include:**
    A Franz Alexander
    B G.L. Engel
    C I.A. Mirsky
    D Wolf and Wolff
    E J.M. Weiss

17. **The following drugs are recognized as useful in the treatment of drug-induced extrapyramidal manifestations:**
    A Ethopropazine HCl
    B Trihexyphenidyl HCl
    C Thiothixene
    D Chlorprothixene
    E Procyclidine

18. **The following statements are true of tardive dyskinesia:**
    A It is commonest in young females
    B The earliest signs are commonly vermiform movements of the feet
    C The movements generally cease on withdrawal of the antipsychotic medication
    D The movements generally cease on treatment with benztropine
    E It is a variety of akathisia

19. **The following workers have made significant contributions to the theoretical and clinical foundations of sex therapy:**
    - A E. Moniz
    - B W.H. Masters and V.E. Johnson
    - C H.S. Kaplan
    - D J.F.J. Cade
    - E Cerletti and Bini

20. **Depressive symptoms that predict a good response to electroconvulsive therapy include:**
    - A Psycho-motor retardation
    - B Hysterical symptoms
    - C Addictions
    - D Guilty ruminations
    - E Delusions of somatic dysfunction

21. **Factors influencing the prevalence of abuse of any particular street drug include:**
    - A Availability
    - B Speed of action of drug
    - C The ability of the drug to cause physical dependence
    - D Cultural guidelines
    - E The ability of the drug to provide symptom relief

22. **The following statements concerning the treatment of alcoholism are correct:**
    - A The Alcoholics Anonymous programme is less effective than conventional psychiatric therapies
    - B Chronic substitution of tranquillizers is a responsible treatment goal
    - C Disulfiram is an effective substitute for alcohol
    - D Alcoholics Anonymous would be more effective if the therapists were licenced
    - E Restoring self-esteem is part of treatment

23. Recognized signs and symptoms of delirium tremens include:

A Profound disorientation
B Markedly increased sweating
C Hallucinations
D Delusions
E Weakness of lateral gaze

24. The following statements concerning international studies of mental illness are correct:

A The Present State Examination (PSE) has provided a high degree of diagnostic reliability
B M. Kramer (1961) reported that the admission rate for schizophrenia was lower in the United States than in England and Wales
C Cooper *et al.* (1972) described the US–UK Diagnostic Project
D The International Pilot Study of Schizophrenia (IPSS) World Health Organization (1973) showed that 'nuclear' schizophrenia does not exist outside of Western countries
E M. Kramer (1961) reported that the admission rate for manic-depressive illness was lower in the United States than in England and Wales

25. The antidotes in column I are recognized treatments for overdose of the drugs in column II:

	I	II
A	Physostigmine	tricyclic antidepressants
B	Chlorpromazine	amphetamines
C	Diphenhydramine	phenothiazines
D	Nalorphine	heroin
E	Atropine	benztropine

26. **The following statements concerning the Stirling County Study and the Midtown Study are correct:**
   - A Less than 20% of the samples were considered completely well
   - B A higher percentage of schizophrenics was found in Midtown than in Stirling County
   - C Over 50% of the sample populations were found to have psychophysiological disorders
   - D Approximately 5% of the samples were found to have affective psychosis
   - E The Midtown Study concentrated on people over the age of fifty-nine

27. **The following statements concerning community psychiatry are correct:**
   - A Primary prevention focuses on rehabilitation
   - B Secondary prevention is aimed at lowering the prevalence of established cases
   - C Tertiary prevention is aimed at reducing the incidence of new cases
   - D Early case identification programmes contribute to secondary prevention
   - E Programmes of support for new immigrants contribute to primary prevention

28. **According to the M'Naghten Rule, to establish a defence on the ground of insanity, it must be clearly proved that:**
   - A The accused is not fit to plead
   - B At the time of committing the act, the party accused was labouring under such a defect of reason, from disease of the mind, as not to know the nature and quality of the act he was doing; or if he did know it, that he did not know he was doing what was wrong.
   - C The unlawful act was the product of mental disease or mental defect
   - D The accused is unable to instruct his counsel
   - E The accused is certifiable under the Mental Health Act

29. **According to Piaget:**
   A Sensorimotor period development is complete by the end of the child's second year
   B By the end of the first month of life, a baby understands that objects go on existing after they disappear from sight or hearing
   C The preoperational period is characterized by the development of the ability to use symbols
   D The period of concrete operations is from age 2 years to age 7 years
   E Cognitive development is a process of accommodation and assimilation

30. **Characteristics of the majority of delinquents include:**
   A Family income lower than average
   B Criminal fathers or siblings
   C Criminal mothers
   D They are the only child (i.e. no siblings)
   E They are of above average intelligence

31. **Recognized features of diurnal enuresis (daytime wetting) include:**
   A Commoner in girls than in boys
   B A higher rate of psychiatric disturbance than in nocturnal enuresis
   C A higher incidence of urinary infection than in nocturnal enuresis
   D A good response to amphetamines
   E A significant association with anxiety at school

32. **The following statements concerning the epidemiology of schizophrenia are correct:**
   A Böök found a high prevalence rate in an isolated community in northern Sweden
   B Eaton and Weil reported a high prevalence rate among the Hutterite communities of North America
   C Peak incidence rates occur within the age range 20–39 years
   D Typically, onset is earlier among men
   E The social class difference is larger among prevalence rates than among incidence rates

33. **The following statements concerning schizophrenia are correct:**

A Davison and Bagley (1969) reviewed the subject of symptomatic schizophrenias

B Schizophrenics have a higher fertility than the general population

C The closer an individual is related to someone with schizophrenia, the higher the risk of developing the condition

D Someone who is a twin is more likely to be schizophrenic than someone who is not

E Children of normal parents, cross-fostered into a home where an adoptive parent has a schizophrenic disorder, have a raised rate of schizophrenia

34. **The following statements concerning schizophrenia are correct:**

A Large doses of L-methionine have been found to cause relief of symptoms in the majority of patients

B N-dimethyltryptamine has been found to cause relief of symptoms in 40% of patients tested

C Friedhoff and van Winkle (1962) reported the occurrence of a compound in schizophrenic urine which gave a pink spot on paper chromatograms

D Slater *et al.* (1963) demonstrated that schizophrenia and epilepsy are mutually exclusive, i.e. they tend not to occur together

E Wise and Stein (1973) described a reduction in the activity of dopamine-beta-hydroxylase in post-mortem brains of schizophrenic patients compared with controls

35. **The following statements concerning treatment of schizophrenia are correct:**
   - A Fluphenazine enanthate has a longer duration of effective action than does fluphenazine decanoate
   - B It is recognized clinical practice to monitor phenothiazine plasma levels daily during the acute stage of the illness
   - C Hirsch *et al.* (1972) found that the relapse rate of patients on active injections was the same as the relapse rate of those on placebo injections
   - D Psychoanalytic psychotherapy is the treatment of choice in paranoid schizophrenia
   - E Behaviour modification treatment is more effective than trifluoperazine in acute schizophrenia

36. **Characteristics of the 'Sick Role' as described by Parsons (1950) include:**
   - A The patient is expected to seek help
   - B The patient is expected to try to get well
   - C The patient is excused normal social obligations
   - D The patient is regarded as being responsible for his incapacity
   - E The patient is not expected to co-operate with treatment

37. **The following statements concerning suicide are correct:**
   - A Japanese suicide rates altered after the Second World War to become more similar to the American pattern
   - B Emil Durkheim worked with P. Sainsbury in London on suicide prevention
   - C Suicide rates are higher in autumn and winter than in spring and summer
   - D Rates for rural areas of England and Wales are higher than rates for urban areas
   - E Retrospective studies (Barraclough *et al.*, 1974) suggest that over 90% of suicides have suffered from a diagnosable mental illness at some time

38. **The following activities are recognized as being of significant value in suicide prevention:**
   - A Ready availability of tricyclic antidepressants to depressed teenage girls
   - B Early discharge of hospitalized depressed patients
   - C Use of ECT in psychotic depressive illness
   - D Teaching psychiatry to medical students
   - E Psychiatric assessment of parasuicides (attempted suicide)

39. **Recognized motives underlying parasuicide (attempted suicide) include:**
   - A 'Cry for help'
   - B Fear of the unknown
   - C Aggression towards others
   - D Testing the benevolence of fate
   - E A wish to die

40. **Recognized predictors of the likelihood of a further parasuicide (attempted suicide) act in an individual include:**
   - A Previous history of psychiatric treatment
   - B Previous parasuicide
   - C Diagnosis of sociopathy
   - D Problems in the use of alcohol
   - E Severe toxicity or self-injury as a result of the parasuicide

41. **Recognized predictors indicating an increased likelihood of a *fatal* outcome of a further suicide attempt in an individual include:**
   - A Unemployment
   - B Retirement
   - C Living alone
   - D Poor physical health
   - E Alcoholism

42. **Recognized features of the Rubella (German Measles) syndrome in infants include:**
   A Cardiac anomalies
   B Deafness
   C Cataracts
   D Mental handicap
   E Specific chromosomal abnormalities

43. **Factors recognized as causing brain damage in the fetus neonate *or* infant include:**
   A Kernicterus
   B Rhesus incompatability
   C Encephalomyelitis from vaccination
   D Maternal phobias
   E Lead poisoning

44. **The following statements concerning syndromes of mental handicap are correct:**
   A In maple syrup urine disease there is characteristically excessive accumulation of galactose in the blood
   B In Niemann–Pick disease there is characteristically excessive accumulation of amino acids in the blood
   C In the Sturge–Weber syndrome there is classically a facial naevus
   D The majority of patients with neurofibromatosis (von Recklinghausen's disease) are severely mentally retarded
   E Hydrocephalus is significantly associated with the Arnold–Chiari malformation

45. **Recognized features of infantile autism include:**
   A Greater interest shown in moving objects than in stationary ones
   B Self-stimulation
   C Obsessive behaviour
   D Echolalia
   E Good interpersonal relations

46. The following statements concerning drug abuse are correct
    A Methadone is non-addictive
    B There is a significant positive correlation between heroin addiction and hepatitis
    C Methadone is shorter-acting than heroin
    D The majority of heroin-using Vietnam veterans were still dependent twelve months after returning to the U.S.A.
    E Methadone produces a stronger psychological effect than does heroin

47. Drugs recognized as causing paranoid states include:
    A Cannabis
    B Amphetamines
    C Chlorpromazine
    D Haloperidol
    E Alcohol

48. The following statements concerning recognized effects of drugs on sexual performance are correct:
    A Phenothiazines cause premature ejaculation
    B Anticholinergics impair erection
    C Heavy usage of marihuana increases libido
    D Cyproterone acetate decreases libido
    E Haloperidol increases sexual activity

49. Recognized features of the phobic-anxiety depersonalization syndrome (Roth, 1959) include:
    A Commoner in females
    B Fainting attacks
    C Good response to ECT
    D Weight loss
    E Specific animal phobias

50. Recognized symptoms or signs of organic mental disorder include:
    A Catastrophic reaction
    B Perseveration
    C Confabulation
    D Emotional lability
    E Memory impairment

51. **Recognized symptoms or signs of hepatic encephalopathy include:**
   A Flapping tremor
   B Slurred speech
   C Mental confusion
   D Coma
   E Extensor plantar responses

52. **The Royal College of Psychiatrists (1977) made recommendations that where ECT is to be given against the patient's wishes:**
   A Anaesthesia should be given by a consultant psychiatrist
   B The nearest relative should be notified after the ECT
   C A certificate under the Mental Health Act should be completed
   D An opinion from a consultant neurologist should be obtained
   E Approval should be obtained from the secretary of the Royal College

53. **Recognized *contra-indications* to leucotomy include:**
   A Schizophrenia
   B Anxiety states
   C Obsessional neurosis
   D Psychopathy
   E Dementia

54. **Recognized features of anorexia nervosa include:**
   A Age of onset prior to 25 years
   B Denial of illness
   C Absence of hunger
   D Amenorrhea
   E Excessive masturbation

55. **Factors significantly associated with poor outcome in anorexia nervosa include:**
   A Male sex
   B Membership of Social Classes IV or V
   C Onset in the third decade or later
   D Married status
   E Persistent overeating with attendant vomiting and purging

56. **According to Cannon, responses preparing an animal to fight or flee include:**
   A Bradycardia
   B Transfer of blood from muscles to gut
   C Constriction of pupils
   D Increased sweating
   E Increased respiratory rate

57. **Drugs which have been reported as being of value include:**
   A Pyridoxine; for depression associated with oral contraceptives
   B Tryptophan with antidepressants; for depression
   C Phenelzine with amitriptyline; for intractable depression
   D Monoamine oxidase inhibitors; for phobic anxiety state
   E Phenelzine with cheese; for acute mania

58. **The following statements are true of drugs taken in excessive quantities (overdoses) in the majority of cases:**
   A Lithium carbonate is safer than chlordiazepoxide
   B Chlorpromazine is safer than amitriptyline
   C Phenelzine is safer than flurazepam
   D Aspirin is safer than diazepam
   E Methyl alcohol is safer than thioridazine

59. **The following statements concerning schizophrenia are correct:**
- A Hoffer and Osmond are orthomolecular psychiatrists
- B Linus Pauling believes that megavitamin therapy is of no value
- C The weight of scientific evidence indicates that megavitamin therapy as currently used is highly beneficial
- D Schizophrenia is recognized by most authorities as being a variety of sub-clinical pellagra
- E Schizophrenia is characteristically caused by faulty transmethylation

60. **The following statements are correct:**
- A Karen Horney rejected Freud's concept of the death instinct
- B B.F. Skinner developed object relations theory
- C Sören Kierkegaard developed the positive reinforcement paradigm
- D Salvador Minuchin worked as a family therapist
- E Lycanthropy is the study of poisons

Paper 8

1. **Recognized symptoms of anxiety neurosis include:**
   A Subjective emotion of dread
   B Tachycardia
   C Palpitations
   D Extrasystoles
   E Chest pains on exertion

2. **Recognized symptoms and signs of anxiety neurosis include:**
   A Exophthalmos
   B Transient vertigo and rotary nystagmus when the patient rapidly assumes a supine position
   C A combination of vertigo, tinnitus and deafness
   D A combination of hypertension, headache, excessive perspiration and palpitations
   E S-T elevation on electrocardiograph

3. **Recognized symptoms of hysterical neurosis, conversion type, include:**
   A Glove or sleeve paresis
   B Abnormal movements
   C Aphonia
   D Sensory disturbances
   E Pain

4. **Recognized symptoms of phobic neurosis include:**
   A Dry mouth and blurred vision
   B Secondary depression
   C Fear of objects
   D Delusional perception
   E Disturbance of short-term memory

5. **Recognized symptoms of depressive neurosis include:**
   A Lowered sense of self-esteem
   B Lassitude
   C Sleep disturbance
   D Psychotic delusions
   E Euphoria

6. **Theoreticians and scientists supporting either genetic or biochemical theories of the aetiology of schizophrenia include:**
   A T. Szasz
   B R. Laing
   C L.L. Heston
   D S.S. Kety
   E I.I. Gottesman and J. Shields

7. **Eugen Bleuler believed the disease process of schizophrenia to be shown as disturbances of:**
   A Alliteration
   B Affect
   C Associations
   D Anger
   E Anxiety

8. **Recognized symptoms and signs of hebephrenic schizophrenia include:**
   A Regression to primitive disorganized behaviour
   B Marked thought disorder
   C Waxy flexibility
   D Disorientation of time, place and person
   E Psychomotor retardation

9. **Recognized symptoms and signs of infantile autism include:**
   - A Spinning and twirling
   - B Constant eye contact with people
   - C Good response to maternal affection
   - D Delayed speech
   - E Excessive interest in pets

10. **The following statements concerning the epidemiology of unipolar affective disorders are true:**
    - A Hospitalization rate is greater for males than for females
    - B Peak admission rate occurs in patients aged 25 to 35 years
    - C There is an increased incidence in lower social class groups
    - D Prevalence is higher in the relatives of diagnosed patients than in the general population
    - E Concordance studies of twins have disproved the operation of genetic factors

11. **The following statements concerning affective disorders are true:**
    - A E.A. Paykel found that undesirable life events are associated with depression
    - B Concordance rates for manic depressive psychosis have been found to be 68% for MZ twins and 23% for same-sexed DZ twins
    - C Genetic evidence fails to support the use of bipolar–unipolar classifications of patients with affective illness
    - D Spitz (1946) and Bowlby (1969) demonstrated that the events of infancy do not predispose to later depression
    - E Monoamine oxidase inhibitors are the safest treatment for most affective disorders

12. **The following statements concerning borderline personality disorder are correct:**
    - A The syndrome was described by Gunderson and Singer in 1975
    - B The syndrome was described by Grinker and others in 1968
    - C States of depersonalization, derealization and dissociation form part of the syndrome
    - D The concept gathers together patients previously labelled latent schizophrenia, pseudoneurotic schizophrenia and borderline schizophrenia
    - E Regression into a transient psychosis under provocation is a feature of the syndrome

13. **The following statements concerning the relationship between coronary disease and personality type are true:**
    - A Rosenman and Friedman have published studies on this subject
    - B No significant relationship has been found
    - C Patients prone to coronary disease have been found to be passive, patient and non-competitive
    - D Patients prone to coronary disease show relaxed facial muscles, slow speech and lack of alertness
    - E Type B patients typically have T-wave inversion on the electrocardiograph

14. **Recognized treatments for incipient delirium tremens include:**
    - A Hypnosis
    - B Electroconvulsive therapy
    - C Sensory deprivation
    - D Chlordiazepoxide
    - E Haloperidol

15. **Characteristics of normal-pressure hydrocephalus include:**
    - A Progressive dementia
    - B Urinary incontinence
    - C Abnormality of gait
    - D Invariably it is untreatable
    - E An obstruction to the normal flow of cerebrospinal fluid

16. **The following statements are true of the treatment of acute schizophrenia:**
    - A Intensive psychotherapy is the most effective part of the treatment programme
    - B Chemotherapy is only effective when combined with psychotherapy
    - C Supportive milieu treatment without chemotherapy is effective in the majority of cases
    - D Megavitamin treatment is effective in the majority of cases
    - E Treating schizophrenia with drugs is immoral

17. **Recognized features of Marchiafava–Bignami disease include:**
    - A Originally reported in Spanish females
    - B Demyelination of part of the corpus callosum
    - C Usually spontaneous recovery
    - D A frontal lobe syndrome
    - E Absence of intellectual deterioration

18. **The following side-effects of phenothiazines show a good response to benztropine in the majority of cases:**
    - A Motor restlessness, fidgeting and pacing
    - B Tremor, rigidity and bradykinesia
    - C Opisthotonos
    - D Oral–buccal–masticatory movements in the elderly chronic schizophrenic patient
    - E Oculogyric crisis

19. **Characteristics of behaviour therapy include:**
    - A A preference for observable phenomena
    - B Prior relaxation training in all cases
    - C Behavioural analysis
    - D Identification of events that follow the target behaviour
    - E Identification of stimuli leading to target behaviour

20. **Depressive symptoms that predict a good response to electroconvulsive therapy include:**
  A Unhappiness in response to a loss
  B Early morning awakening
  C Anorexia
  D Visual hallucinations
  E Weight loss

21. **The following statements concerning electroconvulsive therapy are correct:**
  A It is necessary for peripheral clonic seizure movements to occur in order to obtain a therapeutic response
  B Placebo ECT is as effective as conventional ECT in producing a therapeutic response
  C Any therapeutic response to ECT is the consequence of its power as an 'aversive stimulus' for the extinction of maladaptive behaviours
  D The voltage required is directly proportional to the severity of the illness being treated
  E Legal and ethical considerations are of academic interest only

22. **The following methods of treatment of alcoholism are effective in the majority of cases:**
  A Supervised gradual return to normal social drinking
  B Warnings of death or chronic illness
  C *Compulsory* attendance at Alcoholics Anonymous meetings
  D Analytically oriented psychotherapy
  E Aversion therapy

23. **The following statements are true of physiological withdrawal from alcohol:**
  A Signs usually begin 6 to 24 hours after heavy drinking has stopped
  B Delirium tremens is more likely to begin 48 to 72 hours after alcohol withdrawal than earlier
  C Surgical patients are often protected from withdrawal effects until pre-operative and post-operative medications are stopped
  D Hypomagnesemia is a recognized complication
  E The seizure threshold is lowered

24. **Prognostic factors pointing to a good outcome in schizophrenia include:**
   A Family history of schizophrenia
   B Identifiable precipitating factor
   C Warm personal relationships
   D Insidious onset
   E Withdrawn, solitary, eccentric personality

25. **Factors accounting for past or present declines in mental hospital in-patient rates include:**
   A The combination of penicillin therapy and improved public health practices
   B Fluphenazine enanthate
   C Chlorpromazine
   D President Nixon's Congressional Address
   E A falling readmission rate since 1955 in England and Wales and in the United States

26. **The authors in column I published the studies in column II**

	I	II
A	Leighton	Forty-four Juvenile Thieves
B	H.W. Dunham	The Stirling County Study
C	Hollingshead and Redlich	Social Class and Mental Illness
D	Srole *et al.*	The Midtown Manhattan Study
E	Faris and Dunham	Mental Disorders in Urban Areas

27. **Erik H. Erikson's *Eight Ages of Man* include:**
   A Basic Trust v. mistrust
   B Autonomy v. shame, doubt
   C Adulthood v. latency
   D Oral sensory v. maturity
   E Intimacy v. isolation

28. **In order to be considered competent to stand trial, a defendant should have the ability to:**
    A Know his rights under the Fifth Amendment
    B Take part in the proceedings dispassionately
    C Communicate relevantly with his counsel
    D Understand the dispositions, pleas and penalties possible
    E Challenge prosecution witnesses

29. **The following statements concerning Crisis Theory and Crisis Intervention are correct:**
    A In most cultures, adolescence is a crisis period
    B In Western society, retirement is a crisis period
    C An individual in crisis shows an increased susceptibility to influence
    D A crisis invariably results in unhealthy personality development
    E Regression and alienation from immediate surroundings are healthy coping responses

30. **Recognized features of the hyperkinetic syndrome of childhood include:**
    A Specific EEG abnormalities
    B Excitability
    C Learning difficulties
    D Worsening of the symptoms when treated with methylphenidate
    E Improvement when treated with dextroamphetamine

31. **Effective treatments for nocturnal enuresis include:**
    A Imipramine
    B Chlorpromazine
    C Amitriptyline
    D Bell-and-pad
    E Nortriptyline

32. **The following statements concerning the epidemiology of schizophrenia are correct:**
    A Faris and Dunham found the incidence to be higher in rural areas than in city central zones
    B Higher incidence rates were found among immigrants than among the native born in New York State
    C Incidence is higher among married than single persons
    D The prognosis is worse for those living alone prior to the first admission than for those who had been living in the family setting
    E British psychiatrists have traditionally used a narrower definition of schizophrenia than have American psychiatrists

33. **The following statements concerning parasuicide (attempted suicide) in the United Kingdom are correct:**
    A Rates are higher below age 35 years for adults
    B Women have higher rates than do men
    C Married men have higher rates than do single men
    D Divorced men have higher rates than do married men
    E Rates are higher in Social Class V than in I and II

34. **The following statements concerning the epidemiology of schizophrenia are correct:**
    A Incidence rates among immigrants have been found to vary inversely with the time interval since migration
    B There is a lower incidence rate in the weeks following directly on child-bearing than in the general female population
    C Steinberg and Durell found an increased incidence rate in the early months of army service, compared with the second year
    D Brown and Birley (1968) found no increase in the frequency of significant life events in the three-month period before onset of acute symptoms
    E Birley and Brown (1970) found that discontinuation of phenothiazines had not contributed to the occurrence of acute episodes

35. **The following statements concerning schizophrenia are correct:**
    A Julian Leff has provided evidence demonstrating that Bateson's Double-Bind Theory is a significant factor in the aetiology of schizophrenia in the majority of cases
    B Theodore Lidz and his colleagues at Yale provided evidence supporting the Dopamine Hypothesis
    C Family Theories put forward by Wynne and Singer satisfactorily explain why the patient falls ill and a sibling remains well under similarly adverse conditions
    D Wing and Brown (1970) found blunting of affect to be commoner in institutions where patients were socially deprived
    E Wing and Brown (1970) found a significant positive correlation between social improvement and clinical improvement of patients in institutions

36. **The following statements concerning schizophrenia are correct:**
    A Brown *et al.* (1972) found that relapse after discharge was significantly associated with high expressed emotion of the patients' families
    B Wing *et al.* (1964) found that commencing a rehabilitation course was significantly associated with relapse in the first week of the course
    C An intravenous injection of chlorpromazine and atropine (mixed in the same syringe) is recognized treatment for acute agitation
    D Insulin has a biologically curative effect
    E There is a consistent relationship between severity of extrapyramidal side-effects of drugs and their therapeutic efficacy

37. **Disorders significantly associated with parasuicide (attempted suicide) include:**
    A Hysterical personality disorder
    B Alcoholism
    C Mental defect
    D Thyrotoxicosis
    E Involutional depression

38. **The following statements concerning suicide rates in England and Wales are correct:**
    - A Female rate is higher than male rate
    - B The highest rate occurs below age 35 years
    - C Rate for divorced is higher than that for married of the same age
    - D Upper social classes have a higher rate than middle social classes
    - E The unemployed have a higher rate than the employed

39. **The following statements concerning suicide rates in patients with manic-depressive psychosis are correct:**
    - A Patients treated by psychiatrists have less chance of dying by suicide than do non-manic-depressive members of the general population
    - B The suicide rate of male patients is lower than that of female patients
    - C Rates are lower following recent bereavement than before bereavement
    - D Elderly patients have higher rates than do young patients
    - E Separated patients have higher rates than do married patients

40. **Recognized predictors indicating an increased likelihood of a *fatal* outcome of a further suicide attempt in an individual include:**
    - A Male sex
    - B Age over 35 years
    - C Divorced
    - D Widowed
    - E Schizophrenia

41. **Recognized features present in patients with neuroses include:**
    - A Subjective distress
    - B Independence and maturity
    - C Heightened egocentricity
    - D Increased flexibility of responses
    - E Early morning insomnia

42. The following statements concerning psychiatric disorders in childhood are correct:

A Children who manifest behaviour disturbances at school do so also at home, in the majority of cases

B Girls manifest behaviour disturbances more commonly than do boys

C The commonest defence mechanisms in childhood are regression and denial

D Deprivation of continuous maternal care between the ages of six months and three years of life results in the significant risk of serious personality deficits

E Maternal deprivation is a recognized cause of schizophrenia

43. Diseases of the mother recognized as causing mental handicap in the offspring include:

A Syphilis

B Toxoplasmosis

C Cytomegalic inclusion body disease

D Alcoholism

E Rubella (German measles)

44. Factors recognized as causing brain damage in the fetus, neonate *or* infant include:

A Encephalomyelitis from triple vaccine

B Carbon monoxide poisoning

C Obstetrical difficulties

D Encephalitis from schizophrenia

E Encephalitis from rubeola (measles)

45. Stigmata characteristic of Down's syndrome (Mongolism) include:

A Small tongue

B Large skull

C Low cheek-bones

D Single transverse palmar creases

E Incurved little fingers

46. **Effects of cannabis include, in the majority of cases:**
 A Perceptual distortions
 B Time distortions
 C Auditory hallucinations
 D Euphoria
 E Bradycardia

47. **The following statements concerning barbiturate abuse are correct:**
 A Dependence does not occur in the majority of cases of prolonged use if the dose is 500 mg of short-acting barbiturate daily
 B The abstinence syndrome is characterized by drowsiness
 C Fits are a recognized consequence of withdrawal
 D Intravenous use by addicts is safer than oral use
 E Recognized symptoms of abuse include slurred speech

48. **Disorders recognized as causes of impotence or depressed libido include:**
 A Hypothyroidism
 B Diabetes mellitus
 C Multiple sclerosis
 D Temporal lobe epilepsy
 E Leukaemia

49. **Patients with bipolar affective disorder have a higher incidence of the following than do patients with unipolar affective disorder:**
 A Suicide in family members
 B Compulsive gambling in family members
 C Cyclothymic premorbid personalities
 D Morbidity risk in first-degree relatives
 E Extroversion

50. **Recognized treatment for delirium includes:**
 A Darkened room
 B Frequent changes of nurses
 C Tranquillizers
 D Freedom to explore the ward and surrounding facilities
 E Straitjacket

51. Recognized symptoms of pellagra (nicotinic acid deficiency) include:
   A Dermatitis
   B Dysphagia
   C Diarrhoea
   D Delirium
   E Dementia

52. The disorders in column I are correctly paired with the descriptions in column II:

	I	II
A	Amok:	dissociative state with compulsive imitation of words, gestures or acts
B	Koro:	morbid preoccupation with penile shrinking
C	Latah:	indiscriminate murderous frenzy
D	Windigo (Whitico):	psychotic depression leading to cannibalism
E	Susto:	magic fright attributed to soul loss

53. Recognized *contra-indications* to leucotomy include:
   A Previous suicide attempt
   B Duration of illness longer than eight years
   C Failure to respond to other treatment
   D Tortured self-concern
   E Inability to carry out normal work or household duties

54. Recognized features of anorexia nervosa include:
   A Lanugo
   B Tachycardia
   C Persistent underactivity
   D Episodes of bulimia
   E Vomiting

55. **The following statements concerning anorexia nervosa are correct:**
   - A Patients reduce their distortions of body image as they gain weight
   - B The majority of anorectics show moderately severe obsessional features on psychological testing
   - C The majority of anorectics score as extroverts on the Eysenck Personality Inventory
   - D There is an increased incidence of suicide
   - E Premorbid obesity confers a worse prognosis

56. **The following statements concerning bereavement are correct:**
   - A Mortality rate of widowers is higher in the first six months of bereavement than for married men of the same age
   - B Schizophrenia is commoner in bereaved psychiatric in-patients than in non-bereaved psychiatric in-patients
   - C Prolonged hostility towards the deceased makes bereavement easier in the majority of cases
   - D Loss of interest in personal appearance indicates pathological grief
   - E Increased muscle tension is normal in bereavement

57. **Drugs in which once-a-day dosage is recognized as good practice include:**
   - A Lithium carbonate
   - B Amitriptyline
   - C Dilantin
   - D Doxepin
   - E Physostigmine salicylate injection

58. The following statements are correct, for the majority of patients:

A Chlorpromazine is more effective than lithium in acute schizophrenia
B Trifluoperazine is more effective than vitamins in acute schizophrenia
C ECT is more effective than phenelzine in involutional melancholia
D Chlordiazepoxide is more effective than haloperidol in acute mania
E Pyridoxine is more effective than thiamine in Wernicke's encephalopathy

59. The following statements concerning pimozide are correct:

A It has been reported as being of value in the treatment of chronic schizophrenia
B It has been reported as being of value in the treatment of monosymptomatic hypochondriacal psychoses
C It is a tetracyclic antidepressant
D It has been reported as being of value in the treatment of neurotically determined dysmorphophobias
E It blocks dopaminergic receptors

60. Recognized features of Briquet's syndrome include:

A A dramatic or complicated medical history beginning before the age of 35 years
B Pains
C Menstrual difficulties
D Avoidance of medical or surgical treatment
E Optimism

7 1. TFTTT	15. FFFFF	29. TFTTT	43. FTTFT	57. FTTTF
2. TTTFT.	16. -	30. TFFFF	44. FTTFT.	58 TTTTF.
3. TFTFT.	17 FFFFT.	31. TTTFT.	45. FTTTF	59. FFFFF
4. FTTTF.	18. FFFFF.	32. TFTTT.	46. FTFTF	60 FFTTT.
5. FTTTF	19. FTFFF	33. TFTTF.	47. TTFFT	49/290.
6. FTFTF	20. TFFTT	34. FFFFT.	48. FTFTF	
7. TTTFF	21. TTFTT	35 FFFFF	49. TFFFF	
8. FTTTT	22. FFFFT.	36 TTTFF	50 FTTTT.	
9. TFTFT.	23 FTTFF	37. TTFFT.	51. TTTTF	
10. FFTFF	24. TFTFF	38. FFTFT.	52. FFTFF	
11. FFFFT	25. FFFTT	39. TFTTT	53. FFFTT.	
12. FTTTF	26 —	40. TTTTF.	54. TTFTF	
13. TTTTT.	27. FFFTT	41. TTTTT.	55. TFTFF	
14. TTTFT.	28. FTFFF.	42. FTTTF.	56 TFFFT.	

8

1. TTTTT	15. FTTFT	29. FFTFF	43. TTFTT	57. TTFTF.
2. FTFTF	16. FFFFF	30. FTTFT.	44. TTTFT.	58. TTFFF
3. TTTTT.	17. FTFTF	31. FFFTF	45. FTFTF	59. TTFTT.
4. FTTFF	18. TTFFT.	32. FTFFT	46. FTFTT	60. FTTFF.
5. TTTFF	19. TFTTT.	33. TFFTF.	47. FFTFT	52/300.
6. FFTTT.	20. FFTTT	34. FFTFF	48. TTTTT	
7. FTTFF	21. FFFFF	35. FFTTT	49. TFTTT	M/100.
8. FFFFT.	22. FFFFF	36. TFFFF	50. FFTFF.	
9. FFFTT.	23. TFTTT.	37. TTTFT.	51. TFTTF.	
10. FFTTF	24. FTTFF	38. FTTTT	52. FTFTF	
11. TFFFF.	25. FTTFT	39. FFFFT.	53. FFFFF.	
12. FFTTT	26. FTTTT	40. TTTTT	54. TFTTT.	
13. FFFFF	27. TTFFT.	41. TFTFT.	55. FTFTT.	
14. FFFTT.	28. FFTTF.	42. TFTTF.	56. TFFTT.	

Answers

ANSWERS: Paper 1

T means TRUE

	A	B	C	D	E
1	F	T	T	T	T
3	T	F	T	T	T
5	F	T	F	T	T
7	F	T	F	T	T
9	T	F	F	T	F
11	F	F	T	T	F
13	T	F	F	F	T
15	T	F	F	T	T
17	F	T	T	F	T
19	T	F	T	F	F
21	T	F	T	F	F
23	T	F	F	T	T
25	F	T	T	F	F
27	F	T	T	F	F
29	T	F	T	F	F

F means FALSE

	A	B	C	D	E
2	F	T	T	F	F
4	F	T	F	T	F
6	F	T	T	T	T
8	F	T	T	T	F
10	F	F	F	T	T
12	T	F	T	T	T
14	F	T	T	F	T
16	F	T	F	T	T
18	F	F	T	F	T
20	T	F	T	F	T
22	F	T	T	F	T
24	F	T	T	T	F
26	F	F	T	F	T
28	T	F	T	F	F
30	F	T	T	F	F

ANSWER SHEET: Paper 1 (continued)

T means TRUE F means FALSE

	A	B	C	D	E		A	B	C	D	E
31	T	T	F	T	T	32	F	T	F	T	F
33	T	F	F	T	T	34	F	F	T	T	T
35	T	T	T	F	F	36	T	T	T	T	T
37	T	T	F	F	F	38	F	T	F	T	T
39	T	F	F	T	T	40	F	F	T	T	F
41	T	F	F	T	F	42	F	T	F	T	F
43	T	T	T	F	T	44	F	F	T	T	T
45	T	T	F	T	F	46	T	T	F	T	T
47	F	F	T	T	T	48	T	F	F	T	T
49	T	T	T	F	T	50	T	T	T	F	F
51	T	T	T	T	T	52	F	T	T	T	F
53	T	F	F	T	T	54	T	F	T	F	T
55	T	F	T	T	T	56	F	T	F	F	T
57	F	T	F	T	F	58	T	F	F	F	F
59	F	T	T	F	F	60	T	F	F	T	F

ANSWERS: Paper 2

T means TRUE F means FALSE

	A	B	C	D	E
1	T	F	T	T	F
3	F	T	T	T	T
5	T	T	F	T	T
7	F	T	T	T	F
9	F	F	T	T	F
11	T	T	F	F	F
13	T	T	F	F	T
15	T	T	F	F	T
17	T	F	T	T	T
19	F	T	T	T	F
21	T	F	T	F	T
23	F	T	F	T	F
25	F	F	F	T	T
27	F	T	F	F	T
29	F	F	F	T	F

	A	B	C	D	E
2	T	F	T	F	F
4	T	F	T	T	T
6	T	F	F	T	T
8	T	T	F	F	F
10	F	F	T	T	F
12	F	T	T	T	F
14	F	T	T	F	F
16	T	T	T	F	F
18	F	T	T	T	T
20	F	T	T	F	F
22	F	F	T	T	F
24	T	T	T	F	F
26	T	T	F	F	F
28	T	F	F	F	F
30	T	T	T	F	F

ANSWER SHEET: Paper 2 (continued)

T means TRUE F means FALSE

	A	B	C	D	E		A	B	C	D	E
31	F	T	T	F	T	32	F	T	T	T	T
33	T	T	T	F	T	34	T	T	F	T	F
35	T	T	T	F	T	36	F	F	T	T	T
37	T	T	T	F	F	38	T	F	T	T	T
39	F	T	T	T	F	40	F	F	F	F	T
41	T	T	T	T	T	42	T	F	F	T	F
43	F	T	T	F	T	44	F	F	F	T	T
45	T	T	T	F	F	46	T	F	F	F	F
47	F	T	T	F	T	48	T	T	T	F	F
49	T	F	F	T	T	50	F	T	T	F	T
51	T	F	F	F	T	52	F	T	T	T	F
53	T	T	F	T	F	54	T	T	T	F	F
55	F	T	T	T	T	56	F	F	T	T	T
57	T	T	F	F	F	58	F	T	T	F	T
59	F	F	F	F	F	60	F	T	T	F	T

ANSWERS: Paper 3

T means TRUE F means FALSE

	A	B	C	D	E		A	B	C	D	E
1	F	F	T	T	F	2	T	T	T	F	F
3	F	T	T	T	F	4	F	T	T	T	F
5	F	F	F	F	T	6	T	T	F	F	T
7	T	F	T	T	F	8	T	F	F	F	F
9	T	T	T	T	F	10	F	T	T	F	F
11	T	T	F	T	T	12	T	F	T	T	T
13	F	F	F	F	T	14	T	F	T	F	T
15	T	T	F	T	F	16	F	T	T	T	F
17	T	F	F	F	T	18	F	F	F	F	T
19	T	T	T	F	F	20	T	F	T	F	F
21	T	T	F	T	T	22	F	T	T	T	T
23	T	F	F	T	T	24	T	T	T	T	F
25	T	T	T	F	F	26	T	T	T	T	T
27	F	T	T	F	T	28	T	F	F	T	T
29	T	T	T	F	T	30	F	T	T	T	F

ANSWER SHEET: Paper 3 (continued)

T means TRUE F means FALSE

	A	B	C	D	E		A	B	C	D	E
31	T	F	T	T	F	32	T	F	T	F	T
33	T	T	T	T	F	34	T	T	T	T	T
35	T	T	T	T	T	36	F	F	T	F	T
37	T	T	F	F	T	38	T	T	T	F	F
39	F	T	F	T	T	40	T	T	T	F	T
41	F	T	T	T	F	42	F	T	T	T	F
43	F	F	F	T	T	44	T	F	F	T	T
45	F	F	T	T	F	46	T	T	T	T	F
47	T	F	T	T	F	48	F	F	T	T	T
49	T	T	T	F	F	50	T	F	F	F	F
51	F	F	T	T	T	52	F	T	F	T	T
53	T	T	T	F	F	54	F	T	F	T	F
55	T	T	F	F	F	56	T	T	T	T	T
57	T	T	T	T	T	58	T	F	F	T	T
59	F	T	T	F	F	60	T	T	F	T	T

ANSWERS: Paper 4

T means TRUE F means FALSE

	A	B	C	D	E		A	B	C	D	E
1	T	T	T	F	T	2	T	T	T	T	F
3	T	F	T	F	T	4	F	T	F	T	T
5	F	F	F	T	T	6	T	T	F	F	F
7	T	F	T	T	F	8	T	T	T	T	T
9	F	T	F	T	T	10	F	T	T	T	F
11	T	T	T	F	T	12	T	F	F	F	T
13	T	F	T	F	T	14	F	T	T	T	F
15	T	T	F	T	T	16	F	F	F	F	F
17	T	F	F	T	T	18	T	T	T	F	T
19	T	T	T	F	F	20	T	F	F	T	T
21	F	T	F	T	F	22	T	T	T	T	T
23	F	T	T	T	F	24	F	T	F	T	F
25	T	F	T	F	F	26	F	T	T	T	F
27	T	F	T	T	F	28	F	T	F	T	T
29	F	T	T	F	T	30	T	T	T	F	T

ANSWER SHEET: Paper 4 (continued)

T means TRUE F means FALSE

	A	B	C	D	E
31	T	F	T	T	F
33	T	F	F	F	T
35	T	T	T	F	F
37	F	F	T	T	T
39	T	T	T	T	F
41	T	T	T	F	F
43	F	T	T	T	T
45	T	F	T	T	F
47	T	T	T	T	F
49	T	T	T	F	F
51	T	T	F	T	F
53	T	T	T	F	F
55	T	T	T	F	F
57	T	T	T	T	F
59	F	T	T	F	F

	A	B	C	D	E
32	T	T	F	F	F
34	F	T	F	T	T
36	T	T	F	F	T
38	F	F	F	F	T
40	T	F	T	F	T
42	F	F	F	T	T
44	F	F	T	T	T
46	T	F	F	T	F
48	F	F	T	T	T
50	F	F	F	F	F
52	T	T	T	T	T
54	T	T	T	F	T
56	F	F	F	T	T
58	T	T	T	F	F
60	T	F	F	T	T

ANSWERS: Paper 5

T means TRUE F means FALSE

	A	B	C	D	E
1	T	T	T	T	F
3	F	T	T	F	F
5	T	T	T	T	F
7	T	F	T	F	T
9	F	T	T	F	F
11	T	T	T	F	F
13	T	F	T	F	F
15	T	T	T	F	F
17	T	T	T	F	F
19	T	T	T	T	T
21	T	F	T	F	T
23	T	T	F	T	F
25	T	T	T	T	T
27	T	T	T	T	T
29	T	T	F	T	F

	A	B	C	D	E
2	T	F	F	T	T
4	T	T	T	T	F
6	F	T	F	T	T
8	T	T	F	T	T
10	T	T	F	F	T
12	F	T	F	F	F
14	F	T	T	T	T
16	F	T	F	F	T
18	F	F	F	T	F
20	T	F	F	T	T
22	T	F	F	T	T
24	F	T	T	T	F
26	T	F	T	T	F
28	T	T	T	F	T
30	F	F	T	T	T

ANSWER SHEET: Paper 5 (continued)

T means TRUE F means FALSE

	A	B	C	D	E		A	B	C	D	E
31	T	T	T	T	F	32	T	F	T	T	F
33	T	T	T	F	F	34	F	F	F	F	T
35	T	T	T	F	F	36	T	F	T	F	T
37	F	T	T	T	F	38	T	F	T	T	F
39	T	F	T	T	F	40	T	T	F	F	F
41	T	F	T	F	F	42	T	T	F	T	T
43	F	T	T	F	F	44	T	T	F	F	T
45	T	F	F	F	F	46	T	T	T	T	T
47	T	T	T	F	F	48	F	T	T	T	T
49	F	T	F	T	T	50	T	T	F	F	F
51	F	T	T	F	F	52	F	T	F	T	T
53	T	T	F	T	T	54	T	T	T	F	F
55	T	T	F	F	T	56	F	F	T	T	T
57	T	T	F	T	T	58	F	T	F	F	F
59	T	T	T	F	F	60	T	T	T	T	T

ANSWERS: Paper 6

T means TRUE | F means FALSE

	A	B	C	D	E		A	B	C	D	E
1	T	T	T	F	F	2	F	F	T	T	T
3	T	T	F	T	T	4	T	F	F	F	F
5	T	T	F	T	F	6	T	F	T	F	T
7	F	T	T	F	F	8	F	F	F	T	T
9	F	T	T	T	F	10	T	T	T	T	T
11	T	F	F	F	F	12	F	F	T	F	F
13	F	T	F	F	F	14	T	F	F	F	T
15	T	T	F	F	T	16	F	T	T	F	F
17	T	T	T	F	F	18	F	T	F	F	F
19	T	T	T	F	F	20	F	F	F	F	T
21	F	T	T	T	T	22	F	F	F	F	T
23	T	T	T	T	F	24	T	T	T	F	F
25	F	F	F	T	T	26	T	F	T	T	T
27	T	F	F	T	T	28	F	F	F	T	F
29	F	T	F	T	T	30	T	T	T	F	F

ANSWER SHEET: Paper 6 (continued)

T means TRUE F means FALSE

	A	B	C	D	E
31	F	F	F	T	F
33	F	T	F	T	T
35	F	F	F	T	T
37	F	T	T	F	T
39	F	T	T	F	F
41	T	F	T	T	T
43	F	F	T	F	F
45	F	T	F	F	F
47	F	T	F	T	F
49	T	T	T	F	T
51	T	T	T	T	T
53	T	T	F	T	F
55	T	F	T	T	T
57	T	F	T	F	T
59	F	F	F	F	T

	A	B	C	D	E
32	T	F	T	F	T
34	F	T	T	T	T
36	F	T	T	F	F
38	T	T	T	T	F
40	T	T	T	T	F
42	F	F	T	F	T
44	F	T	T	F	T
46	T	T	T	T	F
48	T	F	T	F	T
50	F	T	F	T	T
52	F	T	T	T	T
54	T	F	T	F	F
56	F	T	T	T	T
58	T	F	F	F	F
60	T	T	T	T	T

ANSWERS: Paper 7

T means TRUE F means FALSE

	A	B	C	D	E
1	F	F	T	T	T
3	T	F	T	F	T
5	T	T	T	T	F
7	T	T	T	F	F
9	T	F	F	F	F
11	F	F	F	F	T
13	T	T	T	T	T
15	F	F	F	F	F
17	T	T	F	F	T
19	F	T	T	F	F
21	T	T	T	T	T
23	T	T	T	T	F
25	T	T	T	T	F
27	F	T	F	T	T
29	T	F	T	F	T

	A	B	C	D	E
2	T	T	T	F	T
4	F	T	T	T	F
6	F	T	F	T	F
8	F	T	T	T	F
10	T	F	F	T	T
12	T	T	T	F	F
14	T	T	T	T	T
16	T	T	T	T	T
18	F	F	F	F	F
20	T	F	F	T	T
22	F	F	F	F	T
24	T	F	T	F	T
26	T	T	T	F	F
28	F	T	F	F	F
30	T	T	F	F	F

ANSWER SHEET: Paper 7 (continued)

T means TRUE — F means FALSE

	A	B	C	D	E		A	B	C	D	E
31	T	T	T	F	T	32	T	F	T	T	T
33	T	F	T	F	F	34	F	F	T	F	T
35	F	F	F	F	F	36	T	T	T	F	F
37	T	F	F	F	T	38	F	F	T	T	T
39	T	F	T	T	T	40	T	T	T	T	F
41	T	T	T	T	T	42	T	T	T	T	F
43	T	T	T	F	T	44	F	F	T	F	T
45	T	T	T	T	F	46	F	T	F	F	F
47	T	T	F	F	T	48	F	T	F	T	F
49	T	T	F	T	F	50	T	T	T	T	T
51	T	T	T	T	T	52	F	F	T	F	F
53	F	F	F	T	T	54	T	T	F	T	F
55	T	T	T	T	T	56	F	F	F	T	T
57	T	T	T	T	F	58	F	T	F	F	F
59	T	F	F	F	F	60	T	F	F	T	F

ANSWERS: Paper 8

T means TRUE F means FALSE

	A	B	C	D	E
1	T	T	T	T	F
3	T	T	T	T	T
5	T	T	T	F	F
7	F	T	T	F	F
9	T	F	F	T	F
11	T	T	F	F	F
13	T	F	F	F	F
15	T	T	T	F	T
17	F	T	F	T	F
19	T	F	T	T	T
21	F	F	F	F	F
23	T	T	T	T	T
25	T	T	T	F	F
27	T	T	F	F	T
29	T	T	T	F	F

	A	B	C	D	E
2	F	F	F	F	F
4	F	T	T	F	F
6	F	F	T	T	T
8	T	T	F	F	F
10	F	F	F	T	F
12	T	T	T	T	T
14	F	F	F	T	T
16	F	F	F	F	F
18	T	T	T	F	T
20	F	T	T	F	T
22	F	F	F	F	F
24	F	T	T	F	F
26	F	F	T	T	T
28	F	F	T	T	T
30	F	T	T	F	T

ANSWER SHEET: Paper 8 (continued)

T means TRUE F means FALSE

	A	B	C	D	E		A	B	C	D	E
31	T	F	T	T	T	32	F	T	F	T	T
33	T	T	F	T	T	34	T	F	T	F	F
35	F	F	F	T	T	36	T	T	F	F	F
37	T	T	T	F	T	38	F	F	T	T	T
39	F	F	F	T	T	40	T	T	T	T	T
41	T	F	T	F	F	42	F	F	T	T	F
43	T	T	T	T	T	44	T	T	T	F	T
45	F	F	F	T	T	46	T	T	F	T	F
47	F	F	T	F	T	48	T	T	T	T	T
49	T	T	T	T	T	50	F	F	T	F	F
51	T	T	T	T	T	52	F	T	F	T	T
53	F	F	F	F	F	54	T	F	F	T	T
55	T	T	F	T	T	56	T	F	F	F	T
57	F	T	F	T	F	58	T	T	T	F	F
59	T	T	F	F	T	60	T	T	T	F	F